RESEARCH INTO
PRACTICE

SOCIAL SCIENCE FOR NURSES AND THE CARING PROFESSIONS

Series Editor: Professor Pamela Abbott
University of Teesside, Middlesborough, Cleveland, UK

Current and forthcoming titles

Psychology for Nurses and the Caring Professions
Sheila Payne and Jan Walker

Research Methods for Nurses and the Caring Professions
Roger Sapsford and Pamela Abbott

Research into Practice
Edited by Pamela Abbott and Roger Sapsford

Sociology for Nurses and the Caring Professions
Joan Chandler

Social Policy for Nurses and the Caring Professions
Louise Ackers and Pamela Abbott

RESEARCH INTO PRACTICE

A READER FOR NURSES AND THE CARING PROFESSIONS

Second edition

EDITED BY

Pamela Abbott and
Roger Sapsford

OPEN UNIVERSITY PRESS
Buckingham • Philadelphia

Open University Press
Celtic Court
22 Ballmoor
Buckingham
MK18 1XW

and

1900 Frost Road, Suite 101
Bristol, PA 19007, USA

First Published 1997

A catalogue record of this book is available from the British Library

ISBN   0 335 19695 0 (pbk)   0 335 19696 9 (hbk)

Library of Congress Cataloging-in-Publication Data

Research into practice : a reader, for nurses and the caring
  professions / [edited] by Pamela Abbott and Roger Sapsford. — 2nd
  ed.
      p. cm. — (Social science for nurses and the caring
  professions)
    Collection of previously published articles.
    Companion v. to: Research methods for nurses and the caring
  professions / Roger Sapsford and Pamela Abbott.
    Includes bibliographical references and indexes.
    ISBN 0–335–19695–0 (pb). — ISBN 0–335–19696–9 (hb)
    1. Nursing—Research. I. Abbott, Pamela. II. Sapsford, Roger.
  III. Sapsford, Roger. Research methods for nurses and the caring
  professions. IV. Series.
    [DNLM: 1. Nursing Research—collected works. 2. Research Design—
  collected works.]
  RT81.5.R4626 1997
  610'.73'072—dc21   96–49631
                                                                CIP

Typeset by Graphicraft Typesetters Limited, Hong Kong
Printed in Great Britain by Redwood Books, Trowbridge

CONTENTS

LIST OF TABLES AND FIGURES

SERIES EDITOR'S PREFACE

It is now widely recognized that an understanding of research and research methodology is essential for caring professionals. However, whilst it is argued that nursing, for example, must become research-based, it is less certain that this is being achieved. Until caring professionals have an understanding of research methodology that enables them to evaluate research findings and utilize them in their own research, the aspiration for practice to be based on research will not be realized. Research-based practice relies on practitioners reading the research literature and implementing the findings in their own practice. It is now also necessary for them to be able to evaluate their own practice and the practice of others. Not all practitioners will become researchers: carrying out large-scale research is a specialized task that requires a high level of training. All, however, should be able to appreciate the research of others and understand how to incorporate research findings into their own professional practice.

This book is a collection of examples of research, all concerned in some way with nursing or the study of health and community care. This second edition has been revised by the inclusion of a classic chapter on smoking research, an analysis of Black women's occupations using census data and two new chapters on research into community care which illustrate the diversity which is possible within a single project. The book was compiled to accompany a textbook on research methods, *Research Methods for Nurses and the Caring Professions*, by Roger Sapsford and Pamela Abbott, but it will also stand by itself as an introduction to research.

Evidence-based practice is now seen as central to the development of nursing as a profession. The chapters reproduced here are intended to illustrate the kind of research that can be done by a small research team or a single researcher – not 'grand projects', but small-scale investigations of theoretical issues or aspects of practice. All of them describe research which was done or could be done by a single researcher, without large-scale research grants. The chapters show a great diversity of approaches: differing emphases on description or explanation, different degrees of structure in the design, differing appeals to the authority of science or the authenticity of empathic exploration. They also show the limitations typical of small-scale projects carried out with limited resources; though each is good of its kind, each also reflects the experience of applied research as it occurs in practice, as opposed to how it tends to look when discussed in methods textbooks.

Part of the target audience for this book is the nursing profession: people taking nursing degrees and diplomas, people taking post-qualificatory diplomas and certificates, and practising nurses who want to undertake research or the evaluation of their practice. For this reason, a good proportion of the examples are based around the concepts of health and treatment. The book is also appropriate, however, for other community and institutional practitioners and trainees – for example, social workers, family workers and community workers.

Pamela Abbott

INTRODUCTION

Our approach to social research methods is one of demystification. On the whole, research is an extension of what everyone does daily in his or her life. We all look at what is going on about us and draw conclusions from it, and when we want to see what something is like we go and look. When we do not know the answers, we ask questions, and we evaluate the information we are given before making use of it. We all have to evaluate our own practice, and very often we come to conclusions about the practice of others. Many of us are in jobs where the evaluation of practice or of information provided by other people is central to our own performance – research in the sense of self-assessment is central to what we do. Many times during our lives we will try out a new way of doing things, or be involved in something new which is imposed on us, and we will form conclusions about its efficacy; that is, we shall want to know if what we are doing works and is an improvement on what went before.

All of this can fairly be described as research. What is formally called research differs from it in only three respects:

- First, when formally conducting research we are expected to call on a body of technique and technical expertise. Some of this is indeed difficult – particularly some of the techniques of statistical analysis – but it can be managed, or if not, then we can find others to do it for us; the techniques are not the heart of a research project, but only aids to it.
- Second, we are required to be more systematic when formally 'doing research' than we might require of ourselves in coming to private conclusions; the conclusions of formal research must follow logically and cogently from the evidence, and both the conclusions and the evidence are open to public scrutiny.
- Third (and this is the difficult side of researching), a certain attitude or kind of imagination has to be displayed: we have to be vigilant at all times for the possible gaps in our arguments and the possible weaknesses of our procedures.

The book falls into three sections. Section A contains three chapters about observation research. The first is participant observation of women in labour and in the pre-natal wards of a hospital, done by someone who would be seen by the other participants as a natural member of the setting, even though she declared her role as researcher. She was interested in what information expectant mothers are given and how they obtain and assess information. The second is Julia Cayne's account of collaborative staff development. The third chapter, by Nicky James, is an extended 'reflexive account' of research which she, a nurse, has carried out on nursing. It demonstrates graphically that research is not a separate thing from the researcher's life, the more so when she does her research in an area which matters to her and in which she already has a role to play. In each of these three chapters the research is closely related to the practice of the researcher: the first and last are studies of nursing and hospital practice by hospital nurses, and the middle one is by a nurse tutor reporting on a learning group for which she acted as coordinator. The point of the work is not just to gain knowledge, but to modify what is done as a result of what is learned. This kind of research is central to good professional practice.

In Section B we look at ways of asking questions. Chapter 4 is in the 'open' interviewing style – learning about a topic area by getting those involved in it to talk about it in their own way and at their own pace. The research is carried out by 'researchers' rather than practitioners, but with practice-related aims – to provide a basis for evaluating government policies of community care in the area of learning difficulty and to explore the impact of official rhetoric and actions on the lives of carers. Chapter 5 discusses the decisions that have to be made in setting out to administer a more formal questionnaire survey and outlines some of the practical and ethical problems which have to be resolved. Chapters 6 and 7 report on the results of a commissioned questionnaire study on community care for older and handicapped people carried out in the county of Cornwall. Chapter 6 describes interviews with and questionnaires completed by district nurses, home helps and their clients, exploring what services the clients receive, from whom, and what the providers think about their occupations. Chapter 7 looks more specifically at the use of *vignettes* – fictional cases – as a way of exploring policy and practice ethically and without intruding into people's lives. The two together also demonstrate the strength of combining different methods within the same study.

Finally, Section C has three chapters, included to illustrate the structure of a research argument, two of them again closely related to issues of professional practice. The chapter by Verona Gordon, on the treatment of depressed patients by nurses, is a true experiment: a condition is measured beforehand, a treatment is administered to a treatment group and withheld from a comparable 'control group', and the outcome is measured; to the extent that the two groups are indeed comparable, differing only in the fact of participating in the treatment, we may fairly conclude that any differences are due to the treatment. The other two chapters both illustrate how the same logic is applied in circumstances where allocation to treatment and control groups is not possible. The Doll and Hill chapter is an early paper from a classic research programme on the connection between lung cancer and smoking, and it describes some of the ways in which this connection was established, using comparisons of smokers, non-smokers and light smokers. Finally, the chapter by Abbott and Tyler takes up common preconceptions about Black people's employment and, by comparison with White women, explores the extent to which they are true of Black women.

One dimension of difference between the chapters in this volume is the degree of structure which is imposed on the research situation. The research task ranges from taking notes of teaching sessions (Cayne) or recording outcomes of a counselling procedure (Gordon), through note-taking during labour and on labour wards (Kirkham) and tape recording relatively natural conversations (Abbott and Sapsford), to systematic questionnaire research asking fairly straightforward questions about an easily identifiable phenomenon or less straightforward ones in a more contrived situation and to structured reanalysis of census information. The 'measures' used vary from records of natural conversation through direct questions of fact, attitude or belief to complex and indirect psychological 'tests'. Some chapters describe just the immediate situation; others survey a difference or a relationship across a population; others have comparison or control groups to strengthen the logic of their conclusions by excluding some of the other possible explanations of results.

Traditionally in talking about research we make a distinction, in terms of structure, between 'quantitative' and 'qualitative' styles. Quantitative research, working in the tradition of the physical sciences, aims at reliable measurement of aspects of a situation and seeks to explain variance in these measures, between groups or over time. Its root model is the experiment, described above, with its control group to which treatment is not administered – the argument being that if two groups differ only in the treatment they have received, then this treatment must be responsible for any differences between them. Qualitative researchers, on the other hand, are credited with a holistic approach, refusing to dissect the situation into measurable 'variables', and with the kind of attention to naturalism (studying the situation as it really occurs, not as it seems when modified by the research procedures) which would rule out 'treatments' or control groups. To an extent this distinction holds true. As we can see from these chapters, however, even qualitative research can be highly structured: the Abbott and Sapsford chapter on families of children with learning difficulties has a comparison group which functions very much like a control group, to distinguish what may be attributed to having a family member with learning difficulties from what is 'normal' in all families. The two styles may also not differ drastically in terms of the naturalism of their measurement; it is a moot point whether it is more natural to contrive to talk 'naturally' to mothers about their problems (Abbott and Sapsford, an open interviewing study) or to get people's views by asking questions which are pre-designed but which would seem the natural questions to ask (Abbott's chapters on the research in Cornwall).

Questions of representation have also traditionally been associated with 'quantitative' research, and specifically with survey research. The Census asks questions of every member of the population, but most surveys take samples and have to demonstrate that the answers obtained from these samples are typical of what might have been obtained from the population as a whole. On a smaller scale, surveys of particular institutions have to show that the responses they have succeeded in obtaining represent what they would have obtained from asking the questions of every member of the institution, if that had been possible, and they very often wish to show also that the institution under investigation is typical of others of its kind. This concern with representation or typicality is in fact general to all styles of research. The experimental treatment of women's depression outlined in Chapter 8 would be of little value if we did not believe that the women who participated in the study were typical of the population of women. Studies of district nurses and health visitors are of value only to the extent that we believe the participants were *typical* district nurses and home helps. The mothers of children with learning difficulties whose views were obtained by 'qualitative' interviewing techniques and are put forward in Chapter 5 are of interest only to the extent that they are typical of that group.

We would argue that what unifies all good research is a frame of mind which has been called 'the methodological imagination' by one author (Smith 1975). Good researchers need to be constantly aware of how participants in the research are making sense of the situation, what it means to them, and also of what it means to the researcher and what he or she may be conditioned to take for granted. This means not just 'collecting data', but long, hard thought about the nature of the situation and the part the researcher plays in shaping and interpreting it, coupled with the realization that the subjects/informants are also interpreting beings, and that the sense they make of the situation necessarily affects the sense that the researcher can make. This process is called reflexivity, and it is not something located in the design stage of a study but continues throughout (see the James chapter for a good example). What is required is intuitive insight into other people's interpretations, coupled with honesty in examining one's own motives and presuppositions. Qualitative researchers tend to be most conscious of the need for this and to place greater weight on it, but it has an equally important role to play in quantitative research. The other aspect of the methodological imagination is the analytic ability to spot holes in one's own arguments and anticipate possible objections to or alternative explanations of one's results, right from the stage of design. Stress on this tends to be more characteristic of quantitative projects, but it is just as important in qualitative research to design a project that is capable in logic of sustaining the kinds of conclusions that one may wish to draw. Thus the good researcher is distinguished from the bad one, and from most of us in our 'ordinary life' mode of reasoning, by a self-examination, an openness to the experiences of others, constant vigilance, a constant questioning of what seems to be occurring, and a constant willingness to be proved wrong. The perfect researcher is therefore an impossible being, someone impossibly self-critical, impossibly far-seeing and impossibly intuitive. However, the researchers represented in this volume have at least tried to be good, and there is much to learn from their mistakes and their successes.

Research may be carried out to evaluate one's own professional practice, or to describe and improve the practice of others or of a whole institution. It may explore the shortcomings of current procedures or look to see whether proposed new ones are any improvement over what went before. It may be aimed at changing overall policy rather than immediate practice, or be built into the implementation of a change of policy, or be carried out to assess the costs and benefits of a policy change. It may be aimed more generally at establishing areas of policy where change is desirable and exploring the aspects of policy or customary practice which may be amenable to change – or at adding to the general 'stock of knowledge', with perhaps comes to the same thing. Whatever its aims and its focus, similar concerns and problems underlie all attempts to carry out research systematically, lucidly and usefully.

References

Abbott, P. A. and Sapsford, R. J. (forthcoming) *Research Methods for Nurses and the Caring Professions*. Buckingham: Open University Press.

Smith, H. W. (1975) *Strategies of Social Research: the Methodological Imagination*. Englewood Cliffs, NJ: Prentice Hall.

ACKNOWLEDGEMENTS

Three of the chapters have appeared in previous edited collections, and we should like to express our grateful thanks:

- to the Royal College of Nursing for permission to reprint 'Labouring in the dark: limitations on the giving of information to enable patients to orientate themselves to the likely events and timescale of labour', by Mavis J. Kirkham, originally published in *Nursing Research: Ten studies in patient care*, edited by Jenifer Wilson-Barnett and published in 1983 by John Wiley, and 'Treatment of depressed women by nurses in Britain', a slightly shortened version of an article by Verona Gordon, orginally published in *Psychiatric Nursing Research*, edited by Julia Brooking and published in 1986 by John Wiley;
- to Routledge for permission to reprint 'A postscript to nursing' by Nicky James, originally published in *Social Researching: Politics, problems, practice*, edited by Colin Bell and Helen Roberts and published in 1984 by Routledge & Kegan Paul.

Four of the chapters originally appeared in journals, and our gratitude should be recorded:

- to the RCN Publishing Company for permission to reproduce 'Studying policy and practice: use of vignettes' by Pamela Abbott and Roger Sapsford, which appeared originally in 1993 in *Nurse Researcher*, Vol. 1, pp. 81–91;
- to Blackwell Science Ltd and to the author for permission to reproduce 'Portfolios: a developmental influence' by Julia V. Cayne, which appeared originally in 1995 in *Journal of Advanced Nursing*, Vol. 21, pp. 395–405;
- to the BMJ Publishing Group for permission to reproduce 'The mortality of doctors in relation to their smoking habits' by Richard Doll and A. Bradford Hill, which appeared originally in *British Medical Journal*, 26 June 1954, pp. 1451–5; and
- to the London School of Economics for permission to reproduce 'Ethnic variation in the female labour force: a research note' by Pamela Abbott and Melissa Tyler, which appeared originally in 1995 in the *British Journal of Sociology*, Vol. 46, pp. 339–53.

We are also grateful to Open University Press for permission to re-use 'Leaving it to Mum: Community care for mentally handicapped children', originally the second part of a longer monograph published in 1987, *Community Care for Mentally Handicapped Children: The origins and consequences of a social policy*. Chapter 5 was written for the first edition of this book, and Chapters 6 and 7 were written especially for the current edition.

OBSERVING AND PARTICIPATING

Introduction

In this section the three chapters are concerned with investigating research questions by looking at what goes on in a situation in which the researcher is participating. (They are all of the 'qualitative' style; systematic observation, in which one measures the incidence of predetermined behaviours, is discussed in the next section.) This is the 'boundary case' between research and everyday experience. The normal way of finding out what is going on, or trying out ideas about what is going on, is to go and look for oneself. The major difference between the research stance and that of everyday common sense is that good research is always disciplined in a way and to an extent which is seldom (unfortunately) typical of our everyday judgements. The two substantive research papers we consider in this section (Chapter 1 by Mavis Kirkham and Chapter 2 by Julia Cayne) consist of reports of observations: Kirkham 'sat in' on labour and people's experience of prenatal wards, and Cayne was facilitator for staff development sessions. The research topics were important for both of them: Kirkham was a trained nurse studying an aspect of hospital practice with the implicit aim of improving it, and Cayne was a nurse tutor trying out a potentially fruitful way of carrying out her job. They do not just claim to report as diarists, however, chronicling 'facts'. They are both properly aware of their impact on the situation and of their intention to 'prove points on the material', and they therefore make every effort to make it equally possible for the opposite to be proved. This is the major discipline of the 'methodological imagination' – to stand far enough back from its own intentions to allow critics the chance to attack them, and to provide the evidence with which they may do so.

The sharpest tool for doing this is *reflexivity* – a process of constantly reflecting on the content and process of the research and trying to be one's own critic. The researcher, while immersed in the social situation, needs at the same time to be very keenly aware of how it would appear to an outsider. He or she needs to be aware of the little things that can determine the nature of the data – interruptions, the presence of outsiders, the injudicious use of a theoretical concept by the researcher herself or himself. Initial introductions are crucial; how the situation is seen by the informants, and therefore what they see as relevant to the researcher, can be determined by the way in which the research is presented by the researcher – or, more likely, by the 'gatekeepers' through whom he or she has obtained access to the situation. How the researcher is perceived by the 'real' participants in the situation – as a colleague, a tool of management, a way of influencing management, a snoop, an irrelevant academic – necessarily affects both the access the researcher can gain to the situation and what goes on while he or she is in a position to observe it.

The interpretation of what is going on is further complicated by the fact that the observer is also a participant both in the situation and in the research. We do not 'record facts' in some neutral way, but make sense to ourselves of the sense which participants appear to us to be making of the situation. This means that the impedimenta of our previous lives are a part of the research – our attitudes, our social location, our preconceptions. It is necessary to put these by and understand the situation in the way that the participants understand it, but at the same time to maintain distance from the participants and feel free to make a sense of the situation which is not necessarily the participants' sense. This is particularly problematic, in terms of feasibility and also in terms of maintaining one's own mental balance, when the situation you are observing is one with which you are thoroughly and professionally familiar and involved. Nicky James's chapter, the third in this section, is an insightful discussion of many of these problems.

Reflexivity appears in two places in the process of research, one visible and one mostly invisible. The visible place for it is in the research report, where the researcher uses reflexive discussion of the research process to demonstrate that his or her conclusions are validly drawn, or to discuss the extent to which validity may be claimed. The invisible but more important place for reflexivity is in the conduct of the research. The methodological imagination requires constant vigilance, constant self-questioning about what may be producing information which is not typical of how the participant might normally speak or behave but be due to something which the researcher has done or some way in which the situation has been presented – personal reactivity or procedural reactivity. One needs to try to see the situation from the point of view of the participants – the research situation as well as the participants' normal situation – and be sensitively aware of anything which might be influencing what is said or done. The reflexive account in the report is offered as evidence of validity; the reflexive process in the research is what ensures the validity of what is reported.

A less emphasized topic in this kind of research, but an important one, is the question of typicality or representative sampling. In a survey asking questions of a sample of some population it would be routine on the part of the researcher to establish to the satisfaction of the reader that the sample is representative of the population, that answers obtained from it are typical of what would be obtained from the whole population. In the smaller-scale and more intense research studies exemplified in this section, however, questions of typicality are equally important. A description of a setting may be thoroughly convincing, but it carries weight only to the extent that we can determine the bounds of generalization. We need to be able to assess whether the situation is unique (and perhaps interesting, but of no importance outside its own confines), or typical of certain extremes, or typical of the middle range of a whole class of similar situations which might include ones that we ourselves will probably encounter. Mavis Kirkham's chapter would be less interesting if we thought that the cases she observed and the handling of information were specific to the hospital in which she observed them, rather than typical of maternity cases and maternity wards. Julia Cayne's chapter would be read differently if we supposed that she was describing nurse students who were unique and that what she said had no bearing whatsoever on groups which we ourselves might join or run.

LABOURING IN THE DARK: LIMITATIONS ON THE GIVING OF INFORMATION TO ENABLE PATIENTS TO ORIENTATE THEMSELVES TO THE LIKELY EVENTS AND TIMESCALE OF LABOUR

Mavis Kirkham

Today almost all women in this country experience labour as patients. Often this is their first experience of hospitalization though antenatal care may serve as a training in the patient role (Graham 1977). They therefore need to adjust both to being patients and to the technical setting of the labour ward.

Technical developments have made possible accurate monitoring and adjustment of the physiological variables of labour. Though the general usefulness of obstetric innovation is much debated, the equipment involved highlights the abnormal and thereby may contribute to the security of staff and patients. The connections to the various machines involved plus the convenience of the staff greatly limit the patient's physical movement and decrease her comfort. Analgesic technology has, however, advanced at a great pace. Epidural anaesthesia has revolutionized pain relief in labour. Yet whilst removing pain it also removes sensation from the area concerned which can further emphasize the patient's passive role. Experiencing discomfort caused by her setting, yet lacking pain and also feedback from her body, the patient has considerable need for information and is better able to absorb it than a patient in pain. Being in an unfamiliar setting and in the care of strangers greatly increases the information she seeks.

There are problems in the transmission of information within any institutional setting. Riley (1977) looked at the structural organization of maternity hospitals in this light:

> The best-informed reforms will not succeed in making hospitals fully humane, since institutions which depend on rigidly maintained hierarchy and strict division of labour among their personnel cannot fail to transfer the results in some form to the treatment of patients . . . the difficulties of acquiring a theoretical appreciation of need are as

nothing compared with the difficulties of *enacting* flexibility within an inflexibly organised system.

The very reasons for the existence of hospitals, the centralization of medical expertise and equipment for maximum efficiency, to a large extent dictate the structure and, therefore, the problems of the patients within that structure. Freidson (1970) looked at the implications of the professional dominance caused by medical expertise;

> the dominant profession stands in an entirely different structural relationship to the division of labour than does the subordinate profession. In essence, the difference reflects the existence of a *hierarchy of institutional expertise* . . . [which] can have the same effect upon the experience of the client as bureaucracy is said to have.

Many studies have shown that communication with hospital patients is generally inadequate (McGhee 1961; Raphael 1969; Franklin 1974). Various reasons have been suggested for staff's failure to give information to patients. These include a view amongst staff that talking to patients is a waste of precious time, the need of the staff to limit their involvement with patients as a defence against anxiety (Barnes 1961) and doctors' tendency to underrate those aspects of nursing care which cannot be measured scientifically (*Lancet* 1970). Another factor is the way in which patients internalize these very pressures. As Tagliacozzo and Mauksch (1979) observed; ' "good patients" withdraw from those on whom they depend and with whom they wish to communicate but whom they do not wish "to bother"'.

Such a situation is documented in hospitals caring for the sick. The changes in maternity care have brought normal birth within this model. The recognition of the midwife as a limited practitioner (Midwives Act 1902) was only possible within the limits set by the medical profession as to the extent of her responsibilities and training (Cope 1959). This left her, within the limits set down in the Act, as an independent practitioner in cases of normal childbirth. As normal birth moved into hospital, the doctors' field, definitions changed. Previously, all pregnancies were seen as normal until judged otherwise, a judgement usually made initially by the midwife. The reverse is now true as all pregnancies fall under medical management and are 'normal only in retrospect' (Percival 1970). By this logic the midwife as a practitioner in her own right is defined out of existence, and the hospital midwives' work during labour is either obstetric nursing or what medical staff define as provisionally normal and are therefore prepared to delegate.

Within such a structure the position of the midwife, despite our cherished legal and professional definition, clearly parallels that of the nurse. There has been little research on midwives and the giving of information but there has been considerable research on nurses in this respect. Manikheim (1979) observed:

> Patterns of communication between nurses and patients reflect this authority/subordinate role. The care recipient has been a passive, dependent model. It has been relatively easy for nurses, having been

conditioned as women, to relate to the passive model and to discourage independence and autonomy in clients. The nurse often evades direct questions from the patient . . . This communication style indirectly negates the nurse's understanding of the patient's condition from the patient's perspective.

Faulkner (1980) described student nurses 'saying nothing to be safe' and ignoring patients' cues. Macleod Clark (1981) described the strategies nurses use to control conversation – avoiding issues raised by patients, blocking talk and using stereotyped patterns of conversation as well as ignoring cues offered by patients who felt unable to ask direct questions. Johnston (1976) found nurses inadequate in assessing the type of information patients required.

Whilst nursing in the USA is different in many ways from British nursing, Sheahan's (1972) stark analysis of the effects of the hospital power structure on American nursing is of relevance. She saw doctors' professional decisions as determining the care of hospital patients and therefore the roles of those who contribute to that care. Power rests with the doctor rather than the nurse and she concludes: 'If power corrupts, so much more so does powerlessness. It corrupts by changing our perceptions of ourselves . . . being too subordinate, too alienated or too weak to effect change.' If nursing is thus constrained by the hospital structure it seems highly unlikely that nurses will feel able to give information to patients which may give patients a potential for decision-making.

Despite this dilemma fundamental to hospital nursing, communication is widely seen as a basic component of nursing (e.g. McFarlane 1980). The structure which gives rise to the nurse's dilemma also increases the patient's need for information. They need explanations about what is happening (Barnes 1961) and need to become familiar with their new setting (Franklin 1974), as well as seeking information about their illness, treatment and progress.

When systematic attempts are made to give information, the results are striking. Research has shown the good effects of giving pre-operative information on post-operative pain and all aspects of recovery (Hayward 1975; Boore 1978). A small study has shown improved nurse–patient communication can very rapidly reduce patients' pain and decrease use of analgesics (Tarasuk et al. 1965). Another American study showed similar pain relief resulting from nurse information-giving linked to patient decision-making (Moss and Meyer 1966).

Such research is clearly of relevance to midwives working with patients in labour in hospital. The woman in labour is well and undertaking one of the most strenuous tasks of her life. She needs to orientate herself to her labour and to her setting as well as to cope with pain. If she labours in a single room she cannot learn from her peers as most hospital patients do, so she is completely dependent upon the staff for information. Her brief period of patienthood is also a rite of passage since labour is the physiological introduction to parenthood. Is a labour spent as a passive patient lacking the information necessary even for orientation an appropriate introduction to the activity and responsibility of parenthood? Though the hospital midwife experiences the same dilemmas basic to her role and setting as does the nurse, she is the person to whom the woman in labour looks for the information she seeks . . .

Studies of maternity services such as those by Cartwright (1979) and Oakley (1980) were conducted retrospectively by interviews. The consistency of their results led me to believe that there was now a need for a different approach. I therefore wanted to see what it was that actually happened during the course of labour which was likely to lead to results of the kind so consistently found in research conducted by means of interviews.

Method

I wanted to see what issues were important to those involved as shown in their actions and words at the time. Observation was clearly the appropriate method. Labour is a definite process which can be observed.

Participant observation (Becker 1970) was chosen as a method of observation which imposed the minimum of external structure upon observations. Ethnographic interviews (Spradley 1979) were used to help place in context the data gained by observation.

I came to this research as a midwife and a mother. But my observations were guided by those aspects of care in labour which the midwives and mothers I observed showed were important to them. Thus my observations and analysis were 'grounded' (Glaser and Strauss 1967) in the experience of those observed as shown in their words and actions.

I sat during most of the labours level with the patient's head about six feet from her and took constant written notes. The question of the researcher's influence upon the research is raised by this method. It arises at all levels of observation and analysis for as Hanson (1958), the philosopher of science, observed: 'People, not their eyes, see. Cameras and eyeballs are blind.'

Though my role was that of observer, I participated in conversation initiated by those I observed. This was of importance in building relationships with them and yielded much useful information.

The people I observed may well have been on their 'best behaviour' because I was observing them. This, in itself, highlights what behaviour is seen as 'best'. The people I observed had more important pressures upon them than those caused by my presence and these were the things I wanted to study. Thus the opportunity to study these pressures at work, plus the relative insignificance they give to the observer, together, make up the great advantage of the method.

This paper is based upon observations taken down in writing during 90 labours in a consultant unit in a teaching hospital in a northern city. The women whose labours I observed were also interviewed postnatally. Eighty-five patients in the same unit were interviewed antenatally. I also observed five home confinements in the same city and 18 labours in a GP Unit in an adjacent rural area. Many of the midwives concerned were interviewed at the end of the fieldwork.

These labours were chosen as normal labours, as far as anyone can tell this in advance. I therefore did not observe women with known medical or obstetrical abnormalities. Nor did I observe where care may have been unusual, for example private patients or staff.

This is a piece of qualitative, descriptive research which does not aim to be statistical.

Findings

The patient's search for information

. . .

All the patients I interviewed wanted information with which to orientate themselves and described their ideal midwife as one who volunteered such information. Mrs 56 said: 'If they don't tell you, you don't know where you are.' I was repeatedly told: 'You need to know'; 'You need to know or you're in the dark'; 'To know what to expect'; 'To know so you're prepared'; 'To know so you're not frightened'; 'As long as I know what's going on I'm OK.' For many women the main thing they wanted of the midwife was for her: 'To constantly tell you exactly what's happening all the time' (Mrs 73). The word 'exactly' was very frequently used in this context.

Some women conceded that 'there are women who don't want to know', but no one included herself in this category. Many women expressed the need 'not to be fobbed off' or said they wanted 'honest answers not the brushoff'. They acknowledged the uncertainties of labour and wanted the midwife to share her estimates, 'even if she's wrong' and especially if labour did not progress normally. 'I'd rather know than just look at their faces', said Mrs 55. 'I was a bit at a loss. Then she said "If the head doesn't turn you'll need forceps." I was glad she said that. I was prepared', said Mrs 20. All the women I interviewed wanted to be 'prepared' in this sense.

Patients in other hospital settings gain information from their peers (Roth 1963). The woman in labour, lacking this source of information, is in this respect, as in many others, particularly dependent upon the staff. The staff are important to her and she is considerate towards them.

In order to be considerate she has first to learn the values of the staff. She therefore shows respect for their expertise and learns staff priorities from their actions and the cues they give.

The admission procedure is in this sense highly educational for the patient. The form-filling usually starts with: 'When did your contractions become regular?' Patients' replies to this question are often quite lengthy descriptions of the circumstances and sensations of early labour. The form requires a short precise answer and the midwife usually fills it in with a remark such as: 'I'll put 4.30.' After that the patients' replies typically become much shorter. Similarly if, after examining the patient, the midwife tells her something of her findings, the patient is likely to ask one or more questions which will put this information into context for herself. If she is told nothing she usually feels she should not ask. The patients I observed were very eager to please and to do the 'right thing'. But their need for information remained.

Patients of higher social class convey to the staff an image of themselves as articulate and clearly used to obtaining information and taking decisions. Their social skills and general manner create an atmosphere in which staff are likely to give information. A student midwife said to Mrs 13 (librarian, married to a company director, ex-city councillor): 'I assess my patients by their intelligence and see what they will understand. Like you can see that monitor's not working.' Several patients of lower social class in the same situation thought the baby's heart had stopped when there was no trace on the monitor but did not like to ask about it.

Patients of social class 1 or 2 (by the Registrar General's Classification), because they will 'understand', are offered more information without asking questions. For instance Mrs 54 (a social worker married to a vet) was told by sister in early labour that a vaginal examination was necessary before pain relief could be given 'so bear in mind that it will take about 20 minutes'. Staff also tended to ask such patients about their perceptions and preferences during labour. Such conversation made it possible for these patients to make decisions and exercise choice.

Patients of lower social class or less 'intelligence' did not receive more information to balance their lack, though my interviews with them showed that they wanted it. They were given sparse information apparently because they were felt to be less likely to 'understand'. Staff seemed to find such patients less predictable or trustworthy within the setting of the ward. The emotional order of this setting was a source of security for the staff which they did not wish disturbed. They were, therefore, unlikely to entrust patients with information unless the patients could in some way set the staff at ease and establish themselves as trustworthy in their eyes. Various tactics were used to achieve this.

Tactics for gaining information

Questions

Questions are the obvious way to gather information. On the labour ward this is not easy. For a question to be asked someone has to make themselves available to answer the question. Patients are likely to ask questions if:

1 The person they are asking has been present for a few minutes and appears likely to stay long enough to answer the question.
2 That person is sitting near the patient rather than standing over her or at a great distance from her.
3 That person is not speaking herself.
4 That person is looking at the patient, rather than the notes, the monitor or a colleague.
5 That person is not actually causing pain or discomfort to the patient at the time (e.g. by doing a vaginal examination or putting up a drip).

These criteria are unlikely to be met on precisely those occasions when the staff learn new information about the progress of the labour (such as vaginal examination). They are also least likely to be met by those staff (obstetricians and sisters) who take decisions about the course of the labour. Patients 'don't like to ask' such people (unless they make themselves available for questioning), because they feel they are 'interrupting' them, as they are clearly 'busy'.

Patients are frequently left feeling unable to approach the senior staff, who hold information, out of respect. On the other hand, the junior staff (such as student midwives) who sit with patients and are approachable either do not hold the information or feel unable to give it, so patients stop asking them out of sympathy with their situation.

If early questions are answered, the patient feels able to ask further questions. If early questions are deflected or blocked the patient soon feels she should not ask questions and stops. Early questions may also be ignored. An unanswered question is socially uncomfortable and unlikely to be repeated.

For the vast majority of patients there are few occasions when they feel they can ask questions and a general feeling that they should not. Many patients said to me postnatally: 'If I'd asked they might have said. But you don't like to ask.' For such women other strategies are needed.

Statements

Statements have an advantage over questions in that a midwife may take up a statement and give information but a statement does not have to be answered. If there is no response no one feels uncomfortable so the patient feels able to try again, for example, Mrs 75 after delivery:

1.37 P: My bottom feels sore. I suppose it's where they cut. [*Silence*]
1.42 P: My backside's hurting. It'll be the cut. [*Silence*]
1.46 P: [*Winces*] It's the episiotomy.
        S: It's not an episiotomy. It's a tear. But it hasn't gone anywhere it shouldn't. I didn't have time to get the instruments out let alone cut.

Statements may also work where questions fail. By the reaction of staff to statements about her feelings a patient can also learn what is appropriate and possible and thus what can be asked.

Jokes

Jokes, like statements, can be used as direct conversational tactics where questions fail to glean the required information. For example, Mrs 72 after artificial rupture of membranes:

P: Is there much water?
Dr: A normal amount.
P: You imagine buckets.
Dr: You've not got that much when you get to term, gets less after 38 weeks and more will be held back by the baby's head.

Similarly a remark by a patient to her husband such as, 'you'll be out of here in time to wet the baby's head', may lead the midwife to estimate the likely time of delivery in relation to the pub's closing time. As well as gleaning specific information, humour can create a relaxed atmosphere conducive to the giving of information on subjects unrelated to those joked about.

Patients' jokes almost always concerned themselves or their husbands. They were laughing at themselves and encouraging the staff to laugh with them. They were not laughing at the staff or the setting. Thus their humour emphasized their humble role and their acceptance of it. This joking visibly increased the ease of the staff. This was shown in increased conversation with the patient, more smiles and more eye contact with her. Patients who joked were entrusted with more information than most patients I observed. Most of these patients were of social class 3.

Most patients, even of social class 3, did not joke. Joking was done more by husbands or by husband and wife teams than by patients alone. Some strategies were confined to patients.

Self-denigration

Some women appeared to use self-denigration to make clear that their view of themselves, and their search for information, was meant as no threat to the staff. Fat women were often very skilled at this. For example Mrs 21 (part of a long sequence of self-denigration initiated by the patient).

> [*The fetal heart monitor is not working*]
> Student Midwife: Let's see if this machine is playing silly beggars.
> P: [*Pulls up her gown to show the wire and its connection to the monitor*]
> SM: You're a right flasher aren't you?
> P: And I've got such a wonderful body.
>   [*Both laugh*]
> SM: [*Listens to fetal heart*]
> P: [*Asks if she can listen*]
> SM: [*Lets her listen with a stethoscope*]
> SM: [*Takes patient's blood pressure*] It's fine now, your BP.
>   [*It was high earlier*]

Other patients had similar tactics of self-denigration in repeatedly referring to themselves as 'a baby' or 'a terrible coward'. Staff varied in the amount of information they gave but always treated these patients sympathetically and information-seeking remarks, linked to self-denigration, were not ignored. Clearly such techniques are not only used in labour, and their development and use await analysis.

Eavesdropping

One of the main ways patients in this hospital gained information about the likely course of the rest of their labours was by listening to the sisters teaching student midwives or medical students. Indeed Mrs 41 said that she had taken an Open University course between her first and second labours to enable her to understand the technical terms involved in this teaching.

This teaching took place over the patient's abdomen (indeed sister often kept her hand on the patient's abdomen throughout) but did not include her. Some patients were told: 'This doesn't concern you.' A few patients (all social class 1 or 2) were specifically included in teaching sessions and invited to ask questions. For the vast majority this was not so.

This teaching could help meet the patient's need for information as to likely eventualities, as well as to the likely timescale of the labour. But because the patient is eavesdropping she is not in a position to ask for what she learns to be put in context. For example, Mrs 65 observed postnatally 'I picked up the result of the examination from the teaching. But I didn't know how many centimetres there were.' (That is, in full dilatation of the cervix, so she did not know how far she still had to go.) Furthermore some patients were really frightened when sister took the educational opportunity to generalize from her case to abnormalities which were unlikely in this labour.

The passivity of this method of gaining information lay at the heart of both its advantages and disadvantages. All patients used it because it was available to them without causing any inconvenience to staff. But it was not designed to meet their needs and could be frightening.

Watching and drawing conclusions

This is in many ways the visual equivalent of eavesdropping. This was used, particularly, to try to work out the likely timescale of a labour. For example:

> Mrs 15: If it was going to be quick they wouldn't have given me the Pethidine.
>
> Mrs 8: They can't think I'm progressing because they brought me tea.

As with eavesdropping the information is useful only if the patient can place it in the right context.

The move to the delivery room was an example often seen differently by patients and staff. In this hospital, patients were put in a delivery room at 3 cm cervical dilatation or earlier. Some patients, when put in the room in which they would deliver, thought that the delivery was imminent and became increasingly disappointed as it became clear that this was not so. As Mrs 65 said later: 'I felt ignorant because I felt I would deliver soon after getting to the delivery room. I didn't know how long it would go on. I kept thinking I was going to deliver soon. I would have appreciated some kind of estimate.' It was clear that Mrs 65 felt her ignorance as a reprehensible state akin to stupidity, not something she could remedy by asking staff for information though she 'would have appreciated' this.

Language

Patients in labour do not have their own language or culture to which they belong. Conversation between staff and patients takes place in language chosen by the staff even if this is a matter of the staff choosing lay terms. For example:

P: I've got a pain in my, er.
M: Your bottom?
P: I've got a pain in my bottom.

Such exchanges were very common.
    In adopting the language of the ward the patient also adopts its values.

[*Mrs 15 is with her husband. She appears very relaxed during contractions but becomes anxious to know how her labour is progressing. After some debate she rings the bell. Nursing auxiliary answers the bell.*]
P: Can you judge how far on I am? . . .
NA: Oh. You're distressed. [*Leaves*]

The patient has learnt the language of the ward and the legitimate reason for ringing the bell. When sister arrives she refers to herself as 'distressed' and her distress is relieved by an injection. In adopting the language of 'distress', and thus doing what the staff expected of her, Mrs 15 stopped asking questions and did not learn 'how far on' she was until she delivered.
    The language of the labour ward is the language of obstetrics which measures the objective progress, or otherwise, of the labour. Such measurements are not usually given to the patient. There is no language, here, to describe the patient's perceptions of labour. In expressing, or simply experiencing the labour subjectively she is, therefore, likely to feel at odds with her attendants whom she seeks to please. When this is so she apologizes.
    Most of the patients I observed apologized during labour. Many apologized frequently if they felt they were not behaving well or were 'being a nuisance' or 'causing trouble' by making requests or simply receiving routine care from staff who were busy. The commonest words I heard patients say immediately after delivery were, 'I'm sorry', usually addressed to the midwife. Clearly the habit of apology comes from life outside the labour ward. Nevertheless, to use it here the patient must accept an external standard of behaviour, that of the staff, against which she judges herself to be inadequate. Staff find apology acceptable. As the anthropologist and linguist Sapir said in 1928: 'Language is a guide to social reality . . . Human beings . . . are very much at the mercy of the particular language which has become the medium of expression of their society.' The patients, 'at the mercy of the particular language' of the labour ward can only apologize. The language reflects and legitimates the power structure of the setting.

Limitations on midwives' information-giving

The importance of giving information was stressed by most of the midwives I interviewed. Their words echoed those patients used in describing their desire for information and showed considerable uniformity and perceptiveness. 'Explain'; 'Explain everything you do'; 'Don't leave her in the dark'; 'Keep them informed'; 'Explain the doctor's action'; 'Say what you're going to do before you do it'; 'Give information to allay fear'; 'Give honest explanations'; 'Don't fob her off.' These things were said to be repeatedly both as what the midwives felt were important aspects of their work and what they felt patients wanted of them. In this context many of them went on to stress that 'everyone is different' so it is important to 'explain at her level'. In practice there are many constraints on the midwife's explanations.

As the patient's conversation is tailored to what the staff find acceptable, so the staff seek in their conversation to please colleagues senior to themselves. The assumed priorities of senior staff, therefore, considerably affect the speech and action of those more junior staff who spend most time with patients.

The presence of senior staff greatly inhibits the giving of information to patients. I repeatedly saw sister explain a doctor's decisions to a patient immediately after the doctor left the room. Likewise, student midwives would explain the results of an examination immediately after the sister left the room. I did not observe any student midwife being told to give information to a patient or being criticized for not giving it. In this sense the junior staff's assessment of the priorities of their senior colleagues appears to be accurate. Indeed it seems to be considered wiser to omit the giving of information as a precaution against saying the wrong thing. Staff therefore learn to block or deflect patients' attempts to gain information.

P: How long does it take?
S: Babies come when they're ready. [*Changes subject*]

or

P: [*In early labour*] I don't know what to expect.
SM: You don't with your first.
[*End of conversation*]

The patient thereby learns not to ask.

Feeling unable to give information, midwives often give reassurance. Remarks such as: 'Don't worry'; 'We're very on the ball here'; 'You're in the right place' are very common in moments of anxiety and are often given in response to direct questions from the patient. Books on communication condemn such techniques, for example Burton (1958), 'reassurance is belittling to the person who has the problem or worry . . . An immediate effect of this response is to block the person from expressing further feeling'. This blocking technique has the further sophistication that it appears to make the midwife feel better.

Midwives seem attached to routines. (Perhaps they make us feel secure?) Although many routine tasks are clearly of more importance than information giving, midwives still want to give information so they often develop their own routine patter for this. Such information tends to be compressed into packages beginning: 'What we'll do is . . .'. These routine packages, whilst they are easy for the midwife to deliver, may not be easy for the patient to digest. Such patter usually concerns procedures which, lacking feedback, are described from the midwives' viewpoint. So points of great concern to individual patients are omitted and the patient 'does not like to ask'.

Other settings

Conversation in labour differed considerably in the different settings I observed.

In the GP Unit, without medical staff, students or inexperienced midwives, the midwives worked as equals on their own territory. They had no senior colleagues to inhibit their conversation with patients. Furthermore, lacking technical advances in pain relief, they had to gain the patient's co-operation by attention to her physical and mental comfort. Conversation and information-giving reflected this. Patients of all social classes were given more information. (They also experienced more pain.) Patients in the GP Unit sought to please the staff but their behaviour could show wider differences than in the consultant unit, and still be acceptable.

Patients at home were on their own territory. They did not use humble techniques for gaining information. (Apologies were mainly addressed to husbands.) Midwives in the patient's home lack colleagues and their relationship with their patient was in many ways colleague-like. These midwives gave much more information. They often gave a running commentary on their actions in advance. Thus the patient was able to refuse a procedure and some did, which was not seen in hospital. Patient behaviour was tailored to standards which she had chosen before the labour and the midwife was informed of this by the patient and her husband. This provided a sharp contrast with the hospital patient's great efforts to conform to the standards of the institution which she had to learn by observation and humility.

Concluding thoughts and hopes

The patients I observed wanted information with which to orientate themselves to their labours and the midwives wanted to give information. Yet despite considerable efforts on both sides the information given was usually inadequate especially for those women whose need was greatest.

In conforming to the standards of the ward most patients sought information in passive ways which could not gather information specific to their needs. Midwives gave information when ward circumstances permitted, which usually excluded just those occasions when information was learned or decisions taken. These were also the occasions when the patient was most anxious to know what was happening.

Lack of information prevents the possibility of patients exercising choice. This may be convenient for staff within an institution but makes it impossible to respond to patient's individual needs, which the midwives I interviewed wanted to do. Passive patients do not 'trouble' the smooth running of the ward but this is hardly a healthy state (Seligman 1975) or a good preparation for parenthood. In this sense it goes against the basic aims of midwifery.

In the strategies they use to gain or give information without 'causing trouble' to the basic order of the ward, there are striking parallels between the actions of patients and midwives. These tactics are not unique to labour but are developed over a lifetime, or career, as ways of coping from an inferior position. Patient apologizes to midwife, junior midwife apologizes to sister, sister apologizes to doctor. Similarly, each observes and learns by indirect means rather than asking questions and thus confessing 'ignorance' and risking discomfort if unanswered. Midwives, as much as patients, lack an appropriate language and in adopting the language of obstetrics, adopt too its values and its limitations. Yet it is these very limitations which ensure the continuation of midwifery.

I believe that an awareness of these parallels alone could do much to change communication patterns in midwifery. The midwife is still 'with woman' in the very words she utters just where that woman's needs are met the least. An awareness of this would not threaten the life-saving scientific progress enshrined in our hospitals but would enable the midwife to 'dissect the fat from the muscle in the imputed skill of the professional service worker and to determine the consequences of each for what is done to the client, with what price' (Freidson 1970).

The midwife's information-giving can change the patient's experience of her labour whatever the setting:

Mrs 70: I don't think pain is half so bad if you know how long it's for.

Mrs 39: I still felt in control, although I couldn't feel anything, because she stayed and told me what was happening and helped me move. So it was as if I'd got my legs. [*With epidural*]

Mrs 61: I didn't know. I had no sense of where I was. No light at the end of the tunnel. It seems infinite and it weighs on your mind very heavily.

The midwife can provide this 'light'. She cannot do this as an individual in the face of institutional pressures. If supported by the priorities of her profession and the emphasis of her education, however, she my be able to give the information her patients seek.

References

Barnes, E. (1961) *People in Hospitals*. London: Macmillan.

Becker, H. S. (1970) *Sociological Work*. Chicago, IL: Aldine.

Boore, J. R. P. (1978) *Prescription for Recovery*. London: Royal College of Nursing.

Burton, G. (1958) *Personal, Impersonal and Interpersonal Relations*. New York: Springer.

Cartwright, A. (1979) *The Dignity of Labour?* London: Tavistock.

Classification of Occupations (1970) London: HMSO.

Cope, Z. (1959) The licence in midwifery in the Royal College of Surgeons, in *The Royal College of Surgeons of England: A History*. London: Blunt.

Faulkner, A. (1980) Communication and the nurse. *Nursing Times*, Occasional Paper, September, 4: 93–5.

Franklin, B. (1974) *Patient Anxiety on Admission to Hospital*. London: Royal College of Nursing.

Freidson, E. (1970) *Professional Dominance: The Social Structure of Medical Care*. Chicago, IL: Aldine.

Glaser, B. and Strauss, A. L. (1967) *The Discovery of Grounded Theory*. Chicago, IL: Aldine.

Graham, H. (1977) Women's attitudes to conception and pregnancy, in R. Chester and J. Peel (eds) *Equalities and Inequalities in Family Life*. London: Academic Press.

Hanson, N. R. (1958) *Patterns of Discovery*. New York: Cambridge University Press.

Hayward, J. (1975) *Information – A Prescription Against Pain*. London: Royal College of Nursing.

Johnston, M. (1976) Communication of patients' feelings in hospital, in A. E. Bennett (ed.) *Communication Between Doctors and Patients*. Oxford: Oxford University Press for the Nuffield Provincial Hospitals Trust.

Lancet (1970) Doctor and Nurse. *Lancet*, 2(7680): 971–2.

Macleod Clark, J. (1981) Communication in nursing. *Nursing Times*, 77(1): 12–18.

McFarlane of Llandaff (1980) Preface to P. Ashworth. *Care to Communicate*. London: Royal College of Nursing.

McGhee, A. (1961) *The Patient's Attitude to Nursing Care*. London: Livingstone.

Manikheim, M. L. (1979) Communication patterns of women and nurses, in D. L. Kjevick and I. M. Martinson (eds) *Women in Stress: A Nursing Perspective*. New York: Appleton-Century-Crofts.

The Midwives Act (1902) 2EDW7C17. London: HMSO.

Ministry of Health (1959) *Report of a Maternity Services Committee*, Cranbrook Report. London: HMSO.

Moss, F. T. and Meyer, B. (1966) The effects of nursing interaction upon pain relief in patients. *Nursing Research*, 15(4): 303–6.

Oakley, A. (1980) *Women Confined: Towards a Sociology of Childbirth*. Oxford: Martin Robertson.

Percival, R. (1970) Management of normal labour. *The Practitioner*, No. 1221, 204, March.

Raphael, W. (1969) *Patients and their Hospitals*. London: King Edward's Hospital Fund for London.

Report on Investigation into Maternal Mortality (1937) London: HMSO.

Riley, E. M. D. (1977) What do women want? – The question of choice in the conduct of labour, in T. Chard and M. Richards (eds) *Benefits and Hazards of the New Obstetrics*. London: Spastics International Medical Publications, Heinemann.

Roth, J. (1963) *Timetables: Structuring the Passage of Time in Hospital Treatment and Other Careers*. New York: Bobbs-Merrill.

Sapir, E. (1928) *Culture, Language and Personality* (1966 edition, edited by D. G. Mandelbaum). Berkeley, CA: University of California Press.

Seligman, M. E. P. (1975) *Helplessness: On Depression, Development and Death*. San Francisco, CA: Friedman.

Sheahan, D. (1972) The game of the name: Nurse professional and nurse technician. *Nursing Outlook*, 20(7): 440–4.

Spradley, J. P. (1979) *The Ethnographic Interview*. New York: Holt, Rinehart and Winston.

Tagliacozzo, D. L. and Mauksch, H. O. (1979) The patient's view of the patient's role, in E. G. Jaco (ed.) *Patients, Physicians and Illness*. New York: The Free Press.

Tarasuk, M. B., Rhymes, J. and Leonard, R. C. (1965) An experimental test of the importance of communication skills for effective nursing, in J. K. Skipper and R. C. Leonard (eds) *Social Interaction and Patient Care*. Philadelphia, PA: J. B. Lippincott.

PORTFOLIOS: A DEVELOPMENTAL INFLUENCE?

Julia V. Cayne

Abstract

A situational analysis had demonstrated a need to help staff within an orthopaedic/trauma unit review past and plan future learning. One way of doing this is through the preparation of a portfolio. An action research project was undertaken to explore two research questions: Is the process of portfolio preparation in itself developmental? If so, what factors influence this developmental process? Development was seen as a process of change indicated through application of the characteristics of adult learners. The action involved meeting as a learning group to explore the process and discuss the problems. Questionnaires were completed by group members to raise issues for further discussion at interview. The interviews formed a summative evaluation of the process up to the last group meeting. Data were analysed through a process of thematic content analysis, resulting in the identification of various categories. These categories were then used to explore the two research questions. Findings suggest that the process itself does influence development by acting as an initiator to reflection on experience. Owing to the short time span and small numbers involved, the project was intended as an exploratory study and as such it has provided direction for future research.

Introduction

As a result of a situational analysis (Cayne 1992) I identified that a group of qualified nurses working in an orthopaedic/trauma unit did not tend to plan their continuing education in a systematic way, or record the effects of their education and experience on their personal professional development. In fact they did not tend to recognize practice as a learning experience. I subsequently proposed that one way of addressing this problem was to help staff identify their own learning needs and develop a plan to meet those needs. In order to do this it was necessary to review what learning had gone before to accredit prior learning and thus avoid repetition.

As the development of a plan to meet educational needs is a major part of the UKCC's (1990) recommendations for the content of personal professional profiles, it seemed appropriate to use this research project as a way of helping the group of nurses to prepare their profiles. There was the additional purpose that profile preparation would become a statutory requirement, and staff within the orthopaedic/trauma unit were well aware of this, although unclear and unmotivated about starting, even though some had already undertaken a portfolio half study day. Initially I was interested in exploring the process of portfolio preparation, in relation to its role as a developmental influence. I also wished to identify and analyse factors which might in turn influence that process.

I have used the first-person pronoun in the writing of this report because I believe that it is an ethical imperative to be open about one's own role in the shaping of events in a project such as this. Webb (1992) points out that the third-person pronoun is used in academic writing to convey 'an impression that the ideas being discussed have a neutral, value free, impartial basis [which] is rarely if ever the case'. DeGroot (1988) further questions the notion of objectivity and proposes that the subject, research questions, methods of data collection and analysis result from the researcher's own personal experiences, values and perceptions. Porter (1993) argues that the interpretations, values and interests of the researcher are, in fact, central to the research process, particularly as nurse researchers are part of the social situations they study. Although Reason and Rowan (1981) do not explicitly advocate the use of the first person, they do suggest that making it clear 'where one is coming from' contributes to making research 'objectively subjective', which is the basis of their 'new paradigm research'. It could be argued that the use of either the first or third-person pronoun in the written report makes little difference to the way the research was conducted. It is, however, my attempt to make explicit my role in this study.

Literature review

The literature review attempts to clarify two key areas: namely, portfolios and development.

Portfolios

The terms 'portfolio' and 'profile' need to be clarified because they are frequently cited in the literature using similar criteria. Portfolios are seen by Knapp (1975) as a collection of information and evidence used to summarize what has been learned from prior experiences and opportunities. This learning can then be made explicit by translating it into the recognizable educational currency of learning outcomes, which can be exchanged, for example, for exemption from units of learning within a course or module. The personal professional profile (UKCC 1990) also emphasizes the need to record learning, whether it is formal classroom learning, or informal learning from practice. The profile is then to be used to provide evidence of professional development, knowledge and competence so that nurses can prove eligibility for reregistration every three years.

Confusion with the two terms can arise because the UKCC (1990) suggests that a profile could be of value 'as a portfolio of achievement', the suggestion being that a profile is a summary of the current three years of practice which can be added to a portfolio. It does, in fact, seem necessary to maintain a portfolio in order to have something to summarize. Owing to the lack of clarity of these issues at the time of the research, I decided to explore the concept of portfolio as opposed to that of profile. There is the additional factor that portfolios are well discussed in the literature.

The UKCC (1990) appears to view profiles as a means to an end, namely a record of past development and a means for providing plans for future development. Others assume that the process of preparing portfolios is in itself developmental; that having assessed one's personal professional development there will be movement towards being able to develop strengths and critically evaluate weakness (Gartside 1990); that there will be development of self-awareness, personal growth and the stimulation of motivation for independent learning (Lyte and Thompson 1990; Walker 1992). Yet there is a paucity of research to support these assumptions. In fact, Miller and Daloz (1989) point out that there is no evidence to support the propositions that 'self assessment contributes significantly to an enhanced sense of self esteem, self awareness and feeling of efficacy', or that 'students become pro-active organisers'.

Oeschle *et al.* (1990), whose work is frequently cited, also reported a lack of evaluation regarding the effectiveness of portfolios. They undertook a summative evaluation, following portfolio completion by a cohort of registered nurses who were undertaking a post-registration first degree. Their questionnaire was used to define the demographics of the cohort, to evaluate the process of portfolio development, and to evaluate the use of portfolio as a learning and evaluation tool. Whilst the published comments of the students do indicate some learning with regard to their own abilities within the affective domain, Oeschle *et al.* (1990), however, emphasized cognitive learning only and stated: 'It must be remembered that portfolio development focuses on documentation of previous learning and life experiences rather than the acquisition of new knowledge.'

Ford and Olhausen (1991) were explicit about their interest in the affective domain and surveyed the attitudes, beliefs and habits of 115 teacher education students in the USA. Their results showed that 91 per cent stated that their beliefs about assessment had changed and that portfolio assessment in their own course played a critical role.

Budnick and Beaver (1984) reported on their own experiences with portfolios, used as a way of gaining exemption from various units of learning, within their post-registration nursing degree. They reported that: 'portfolios provided an opportunity to review, reconfirm and document our strengths, skills and knowledge'.

They also reported a number of drawbacks. These were: the conversion of terminology from the familiar to the academic, the disadvantages of those who lacked writing skills because credit was awarded on the basis of a written presentation, difficulties in obtaining documented proof, and the lack of guidelines for evaluation which meant that assessment was dependent on the attitudes of the reviewer. The situation described by Budnick and Beaver (1984) where there is a lack of guidelines for assessment seems to parallel the current situation regarding the assessment of portfolios for registration. Certainly, Glen and Hight (1992) emphasize the need for the development and assessment of portfolios based on clear criteria.

Three of the key areas identified by Marsh and Lasky (1984) were used in this study as the basis of a framework for portfolio design. The three key areas utilized were:

1 A summary of experiences similar to a detailed curriculum vitae.
2 A narrative which includes reflection on experience with clarification of learning.
3 Documented evidence to support the areas of personal professional development mentioned in the previous two areas.

Development

A central theme of development, whether concerned with biological and cognitive processes or behaviour, is change (Atkinson *et al.* 1990). Some changes can arise from and perpetuate existing patterns of life, whilst other life events can actually disrupt those patterns (Rogers 1992). On the one hand, development can be a progressive, continuous process emanating from past experiences. On the other, it can arise from a change in direction owing to an intentional intervention through change agency. Change may effect further change, for example self-directed learning, after the initiative ends (Rogers 1992). Thus an initiative such as portfolio preparation could be viewed as a spur for nudging people into a process of development, by facilitating the evolution of self-directed learning. It is the beginning of a process rather than an end in itself which will continue after the initial intervention ends, although in the case of nursing the spur will be repeated every three years, because of the requirement to reregister.

Overall, it seems that portfolios are being proposed not only to inform but to transform the person. The notion of personal transformation through education (in this case portfolio preparation) is based on several overlapping themes. The first is the belief that personal and professional development are one and the same. As Barber (1989) so eloquently states:

> Personal development cannot be separated from professional development; each rests upon the other. Show me how well you share of yourself, understand your own personal processes and are able to communicate this to others, and I'll know how good or bad your nursing care is.

The personal development of nurses and the experiences which have created the person directly influence their professional role and subsequently the nursing care they deliver. In this sense, development includes self-awareness, intrapersonal and interpersonal processes.

Secondly the characteristics arising from personal professional development resemble Knowles's (1990) characteristics of adult learners. These are: awareness of self-concept, the recognition and valuing of personal experiences in relation to learning, readiness to learn related to social and role competence and the ability to be proactive and problem-solving. It is claimed that these characteristics develop during and following portfolio preparation (Gartside 1990; Lyte and Thompson 1990; Walker 1992) and that it is the very values associated with adult learning which underpin the concept of portfolio (Lambeth *et al.* 1989; Glen and Hight 1992). It is worth noting that perhaps not everyone has well developed 'adult learning' tendencies but rather these qualities are something to be nurtured and developed.

Thirdly, androgogy, like a student-centred approach to learning, is based on the premise that individuals have an innate tendency for self-direction and growth given a facilitative climate (Knowles 1978, 1990; Rogers 1983). The facilitative approach utilized in this project could therefore be seen to have a bearing on the outcome of the venture. Effective helping behaviour can itself enable learners to engage in the process of learning (Heron 1989).

Research questions

It was claimed in the literature that preparing portfolios would somehow help provide the impetus for the personal professional development of individuals involved. I wished to explore these claims and what it was about preparing a portfolio that influenced the process. Two research question therefore evolved:

1 Is the process of portfolio preparation in itself developmental?
2 If so, what factors influence this developmental process?

The focus of this project was on actually 'doing' rather than simply talking about 'how to do' portfolios, through a co-operative endeavour. An underlying aim was that the project would have some benefit for the unit as well as for my own learning process. Reason and Marshall's (1988) view of research seemed a particularly apposite one in that research is seen as part of the researchers' own personal process, as a way of enabling a community of people to act effectively in their world and as contributing to the body of knowledge.

Methodology

Theoretical framework

The validity of qualitative research approaches is concerned with analytical rather than enumerative induction, and inferences are made to demonstrate theoretical principles rather than to make generalizations about the population (Kent and Maggs 1992). In turn, the 'validity of the analysis depends on an appropriate theoretical framework' (Mitchell, cited by Kent and Maggs 1992). Having undertaken the literature review I realized that there were several strands within the project which were based on the same underlying principles. The three strands were: adult learning (Knowles 1978, 1990; Rogers 1983; Heron 1989), the developmental process (Rogers 1992), and the process of action research (Lewin 1946).

The common underlying principles were synthesized to form a framework which would guide the study as follows:

1 The facilitation of learning and the action research process require democratic and co-operative interventions.
2 The valuing of, and reflection on, experience enable the development of both group members and teacher/researcher through the experiential learning process.
3 Learning, development and action research are viewed as instruments of change.
4 The solving of problems that have a real world focus is necessary for adult learning and is the essence of action research.

The above principles guided the project, notably in the following areas: (a) the choice of research design and the research process itself, (b) the facilitation process, including the selection of group members, (c) methods of data collection, and (d) data analysis.

Research design

Action research was chosen as the research design. This was because it is a way of studying issues in democratic and participative ways (Lewin 1946). Stenhouse (1975) believed that researchers and the researched should participate in the research process rather than the former simply observe the latter. McNiff (1988) proposes action research as the means by which teachers as researchers can reflect on and improve their own practice. Viewed in these ways, action research becomes research for me (my development from student teacher to nurse tutor) and research for us, through the learning process (group members), as outlined by Reason and Marshall (1988). Thus by working with learners the teacher as researcher is better able to understand their world, the meaning it has for them and the specific context of the problem (Cohen and Manion 1989). Consequently, through continuous evaluation the teacher can monitor and modify the learning and research processes as issues arise.

Selection of group members and facilitation process

I hoped to set up a learning group composed of nursing staff from the orthopaedic/trauma unit. As a tutor student within this unit I wished to undertake a project that would be felt to have some use for both the individuals and the unit. The unit manager and ward sisters were approached and permission given for the project, despite some opposition from sisters who saw the project as draining their already overstretched resources. Several saw the project as potentially beneficial and they were very supportive. There was agreement that group members would be qualified nurses who, the sisters felt, would be able to help other staff develop portfolios. The vagaries of the off duty would, however, determine who was on an early shift on a regular basis on Friday mornings. In the event, the only common criteria for selection were that the portfolio group members were qualified nurses who worked on Friday mornings.

In a way these criteria do reflect the real world, because all nurses regardless of experience and abilities will be required to prepare their portfolios. Limitations of time and availability are characteristics of convenience sampling (Field and Morse 1985). This form of non-probability sampling is particularly appropriate for exploratory studies where generalization to the population is not intended. Within the unit there were six wards, the accident and emergency department and fracture clinic. Owing to one ward closure and staffing levels on another, six people were nominated to attend the one-hour sessions. We met on five occasions over a two-month period to explore the process of portfolio preparation and discuss the problems. At intervals throughout this period group members were offered the chance to withdraw from the study, although none did.

Prior to the first meeting I was aware that trust in groups can initially be low (Jaques 1984) and there is a need to set up a contract about the research agenda with the group (Kent and Maggs 1992). I therefore planned and structured the first session hierarchically (Heron 1989) and set out a framework for developing a portfolio for the group, based on the three key areas described earlier. The rest of the group meetings were to be focused on problems raised about portfolios by the group. I could not therefore plan these sessions in a conventional way and found the modes and dimensions of Heron's (1989) model of facilitation to be an invaluable working guide, which helped me to respond appropriately to the group's needs.

Data collection and analysis

Data were collected using various methods to gain different perspectives of the process of portfolio preparation, its possible developmental effects and factors influencing the process. Triangulation and corroboration, when used in the qualitative paradigm, involve checking propositions either with various methodological tools or with other group members, to improve validity and reliability (Guba and Lincoln 1981) thus giving a 'more full and rounded picture' (Webb 1989). The various methodological tools were: the keeping of field notes as a participant observer (of group sessions), the taping of group sessions, and taped interviews following an exploratory questionnaire. The checking of propositions by group members was done by inviting each individual to comment on a written draft of the findings. At this time, an offer to withdraw information was made in writing.

Table 2.1 To demonstrate the process of developing non-standardized, structured interview schedules: Raising issues through the open-ended questions in the questionnaire and relating them to the research questions

Question on questionnaire	Answer	Issues raised	Questions for interview	Rationale
Why did you want to develop your portfolio?	To comply with new regulations which I believe to be coming into force.	Complying with new regulations.	How did you think compiling a portfolio would help with this?	To clarify issue and understanding of 'new regulations'.
			Do you now think there are other reasons for doing a portfolio? . . . What are they?	Related to Q1 – to see if process has changed this.
			What has made you change your mind?	Related to Q2 – to find out what has influenced possible change.
What has been useful about developing your portfolio?	I am so worried about failure I don't even try.	Fear of failure.	Could you explain what you meant by this?	Having raised what is on top, need to clarify her perspective.
			What is it about doing your portfolio that has raised this issue for you?	Related to Q2 – to find out what has helped this realization.
			You have put this under 'useful'; in what way has it been useful to have this issue raised?	Related to Q1 – recognition of own development.
What has been difficult about developing your portfolio?	It appears very subjective in places and I am not sure how valid this is.	Appears subjective, unsure how valid this is.	Could you explain what you meant by this? Clarify subjective, clarify valid. What places particularly?	To gain understanding of her perspective and meaning.
			Do you think it is difficult to write about yourself? Why do you think this is so?	Related to Q2 – to see how and why this is a difficulty.
			Although this is a difficult area do you think it may be useful too?	To see if she has gained anything from this even though it is difficult – Q1.

In the event, the tapes of the group sessions were not transcribed and analysed because too much data were generated for the scope of this project. I did, however, listen to and use the tapes to check the accuracy of my field notes. The field notes were transcribed into brief process notes using Lewin's (1946) cycle of planning/replanning, acting, observing and reflecting. These notes were used to link my perspective with that of the group when writing up the report. The group members' perspective was explored initially through a questionnaire submitted after the last group meeting. The questionnaire was composed of open-ended questions and the responses were then used to develop non-standardized, structured interview schedules based on the emergent trends (McNiff 1988). Table 2.1 clarifies this process and sets out how the interview questions were linked to the research questions.

Five out of six interviews were successfully taped and transcribed in full. Although the recording of the sixth interview was unsuccessful my field notes for the session were used. The transcribing helped both to increase my familiarity with the data and to enable thematic, content analysis to be undertaken (Field and Morse 1985; Burnard 1991). Having completed this process, 19 categories were generated. Some categories were similar to others and two or more could be subsumed, thus becoming properties within the higher order category. Others could be combined to form new categories. Through this process of data reduction (Glaser and Strauss 1967; Burnard 1991) six categories finally emerged. These were:

1 Reflection on the experience of compiling a portfolio
2 Reasons for doing a portfolio
3 Compiling the content of portfolios
4 The effect of others
5 Time
6 Finishing.

Findings

The theoretical framework which guided the study was also utilized in the development of a tool for checking the validity of findings (Table 2.2). The findings, within the six categories above, were subsequently compared to the criteria within that tool. Everyone in the group talked about the way compiling their portfolio had made them think, reflect or look back on various aspects of their nursing practice. The questions are: Was there actually reflection and if so what influenced it?

Category 1, reflection on the experience, most clearly answers these questions and provides both evidence of reflection on experience and the effect of the lack of valuing of experience, as learning. The other five categories are summarized to show their influence on the process of portfolio preparation. The individual interviews provide the main source for the findings, unless otherwise indicated.

Table 2.2 Tool for validation of findings, to indicate development

Criteria for validation of findings

Self-concept
The adult learners see themselves as capable of self-direction and desire others
   to see them in that way
Maturity is therefore the capacity to be self-directing
There is realization that studying and learning are an integral part of life
As a result there is recognition of the influence of one life role on another
Experience
To an adult, experience is the person, rather than something that has happened
   to them
Adults define who they are in terms of their experience
As a result, adults recognize the value of their experience
Readiness to learn
Adult developmental tasks increasingly move towards competence in their life
   roles
Readiness to learn is often associated with moving from one developmental
   stage to another
Adults can best identify, for themselves, whether they are ready to learn and
   therefore whether they wish to be taught
Problem solving
Adults view learning as the means to helping them solve current life problems
   rather than as the accumulation of knowledge for future use
Adults are therefore motivated to learn something relevant to their life
   situations
The most potent motivators are from self:
   Motivators: job satisfaction, self-esteem, quality of life
   Blocks to motivation: negative self-concept, inaccessibility of opportunity or
      resources, time constraints, programmes which violate the principles of
      adult learning
Learning as a lifelong process
There is the recognition of and ability to cope with the constant change
   process involved in learning.

Adapted from: Tough (1979), Rogers (1983), Knowles (1990)

Reflection

Reflection is that stage of the experiential learning cycle (Kolb 1984)
concerned with engaging in critical observation about experience, including input in the form of dialogue or other material such as that gained
from reading (Rogers 1992). Reflection is in itself a complex process, as
can be seen from Boyd and Fales's definition:

> the process of creating and clarifying the meaning of experience
> (present or past) in terms of self (self in relation to self and self in
> relation to the world). The outcome of the process is changed concep-
> tual perspective. The experience that is explored and examined to
> create meaning focuses around or embodies a concern of central
> importance to self.
>
> (Boyd and Fales 1983)

When viewed in this way the concept of reflection, as a process leading to changed perceptual perspective, echoes the process of personal change, leading to reinterpretation of personal, social and occupational roles through exploration of the affective, cognitive and psychomotor domains (Brookfield 1986). Jarvis (1987) argues that awareness of a separation between one's life history and current and future experience initiates learning. Reflection is the ability to learn from this gap through questioning, rather than simply taking it for granted. As group members talked about their experience of preparing a portfolio they demonstrated varying degrees of awareness of, and learning from, past experiences.

Helen, for example, was hoping that her portfolio would provide her with some ideas for where she should go next in her career. This was not happening and she felt disappointed and frustrated. Although there was awareness of something bothering her, she could not pin it down. Boyd and Fales's (1983) research, which was used also by Miller (1992) as an indicator of reflection, recognizes this as an early stage of reflection which they term 'a sense of inner discomfort'.

> I thought that because it gives you – really I suppose, a chance for reflection over everything, to sort of, I don't know, perhaps categorize what you have done and what you haven't done, what you need to do. But and, you feel that it ought to come out with, what I need to do now is this. And when you don't come out with anything specific, as such, well I thought what I can do but nothing specific, it doesn't know what to do. It feels like nothing's achieved.
>
> Helen

Whilst she had spent time thinking about her portfolio she had not made much headway with the writing because of her need to get it right, rather than just write down her spontaneous thoughts. Possibly the compulsory nature of portfolios in nursing was inhibiting free expression, which is the cornerstone of Walker's (1985) advice for keeping a portfolio. He further suggests that indecision about starting a portfolio needs to be overcome by allowing the writing to flow and then reflecting on it. Until Helen could actually 'sit down and start' as described by several others, she may not be able to move on through the process.

Others were aware of the nature of a problem and its relevance to themselves. They described how completing their portfolio had made them face up to difficulties in practice. Margaret explained how resistant to change the ward she works on is and how she has come to face that and realize how it is affecting her confidence in her ability to develop further (field notes following interview). Sarah also realized how her own specialist skills were not being used, particularly in an area where they could be utilized to improve patients' safety.

> I've, I mean I feel that I've got a lot of resources but people just don't use me as a resource. Not at all. Um, I find that frustrating. Um, and I think well if the knowledge is there well use it and I think that if I could pull out from my own, especially as I'm not a keen teacher, I'm not because I don't – I, you know, really I don't think I get my point across. But I think that if I could – I see so many different

things and – I just feel they're endangering patients. Then if I could pull some teaching bits together – um – from all the bits and bobs that I've done, then – then it's – then you're a resource, aren't you.

Sarah

A significant aspect of reflective learning is the ability to question one's self-image (Brookfield 1986), which is linked to the notion of self-concept. This is something which was happening for Catherine. She had been reviewing her standards of care and her role, particularly in relation to how patients and junior staff see her. She explained her standards thus:

Well, all standards that are required in the policies. You know the standards of um – looking at your work, making sure your work is correct. Making sure you give the right evaluation of things to patients, and the right, um, example to junior staff, like people that come down on the ONC [ENB 219] course. Helping them as well. Helping and teaching them. All those sorts of areas. That's what, um, made me think about them, you know. And I think, well you know, how do people see me as a person? You know how you see yourself. I don't know how you see me and this is what I sort of analyse. How do they see me as a person? As a senior nurse in that department and how do they see me living up to that role that I have?

Catherine

Another significant indicator of reflection is when learners 'reinterpret their current and past behaviours from a new perspective' (Brookfield 1986), something Mezirow (1990) calls 'perspective transformation'. Libby talked about her lack of confidence as an enrolled nurse and how she would 'shy away from things'. By reviewing the past she realizes how her learning has changed and how she can face something from the past 'head on'. She described how she has come to view being an enrolled nurse.

Its come from the last couple of months because – being an enrolled nurse to me always had a bit of a stigma attached to it, you know. Um, I went in expecting to be a bedside nurse, found out there was no way I was a bedside nurse. I was just getting used as all kinds of other things. Um – and having the confidence to sit down and think, yeah, well it was good to be an enrolled nurse. I learned this, this and this from it. Rather than sort of thinking, I can't wait to be a staff nurse. Now I am a staff nurse I can reflect on what I have learnt as an enrolled nurse. Now I've got rid of that stigma of being an enrolled nurse . . . I can certainly empathize with other members of staff, auxiliaries and ENs, because I've been there. Because I hadn't thought of that before.

Libby

As a result of the increase in confidence, derived from her role change from an enrolled nurse to a registered nurse, Libby had been able to learn from her experiences: by identifying and attempting to fill the gaps in her knowledge (cognitive domain), and by coming to value her previous role whilst recognizing its limitations (affective domain). This is linked with Knowles's (1990) proposition that moving from one developmental stage to another is a particular stimulant of readiness to learn.

The theme running through reflection as represented here, is that of recognizing and fulfilling a disjuncture between past and present experience and future direction, summarized by Knowles (1990) as a need-to-know. Reflection is thus a doubly potent tool for learning because not only has the gap been recognized; it has been recognized by the individuals themselves. Adults are best motivated by something they perceive as meaningful to their own life situations (Knowles 1990).

Valuing experience

Reflection is not concerned with just being thoughtful, but about turning thoughts about experiences in practice into learning (Jarvis 1992; Rogers 1992). The belief that the technical–rational type of knowledge is of the only importance can, however, lead to the devaluing of experience as knowledge (Powell 1989). Subsequently learning from experience, which Schön (1987) terms 'reflection on action', is not attempted. An essential factor influencing the process of reflection was the extent to which experience was recognized as a valuable learning opportunity.

There was evidence that courses were initially seen as the only or main source of learning, as opposed to experience gained in practice, resulting in the devaluing of practice experience. Despite going on a portfolio study day in July 1992, the main emphasis of portfolios for Janet was as a record of study days and courses.

> I mean we had to get like, um, certificates photocopied, they said to photocopy them. Easier than using originals. Um, and like if you attended study days to get the attendance form signed. So we had to do that. I knew we could put, like the teaching packs that we'd done, we could put those in. Um, so although I hadn't gathered all that, I had in my mind that that's what would go in, I had got some of the certificates photocopied. And I've got a list of lectures as well, study days.
>
> Janet

Catherine believed that because she had undertaken no courses she had little to put into a portfolio. This was an ongoing theme in our group discussions (field notes from three group meetings) and something that Catherine had obviously thought about.

> Well, when you look at the job that I do, the uh, responsibility that I have and then when I started doing the portfolio and I thought, oh what did I embark on this for, you know? Because I thought I had nothing to offer, only a little tiny piece, you know, and you kept saying it's your experience. Don't think about what you've done [courses] but think of the experience and I went away and thought about that. And I thought about my skills, and I thought about the way I help other people with these skills. And although I'd been doing it anyway I wasn't aware that I'd been doing it and it became, made me become aware of these things that I was doing. To see that

I was of benefit to other people whereas I thought I wasn't. I thought
I was useless.

Catherine

The realization of just how much experience she had and how she took
it for granted came to Sarah once she started compiling her portfolio.

When I sat down, got everything out, as I said to you the other day,
and spread it all out on a table, well there's just piles of it and you
don't realize how much there is to all pull together. And listening to
one of the other girls, well they keep saying they've got no paper
qualifications – um. If I still took away my paper qualifications there
would still be an awful lot to home in on. And I can't see even if you
haven't got the paper, it doesn't really, well it doesn't really matter.
And also I think you can question, you know, well what you have
done and where you need to go and where there is a gap.

Sarah

For Libby, reviewing the past led to learning from experience, in the
form of 'reflection-on-action' (Schön 1987). As a student nurse, undergoing enrolled nurse training, the responsibility for undertaking a difficult
and dangerous procedure had been left by the sister and doctor to Libby.

I remember one episode of, um, as a student, being told to pass an
NG [naso-gastric] tube on a gentleman that was an alcoholic, and at
that time I didn't understand about oesophageal varices, etc. Um, and
I put this NG tube down and of course he bled and bled and bled . . .

Libby

Reviewing the past had led to learning in both the cognitive and affective domains. Libby had recognized that her limited knowledge of medical nursing stemmed from her experiences as a student, and had started
visiting the library to read up on aspects of medical nursing. She also said
that by identifying the problem it had 'made it a little bit better' and it
had altered the way in which she viewed herself as a nurse.

I used to shy away from things, um – I'm only an enrolled nurse, I
don't need to know that. But now I've changed a lot and I do need
to know. I need to know as much as I possibly can.

Libby

The devaluing of experience is synonymous with devaluing the self
because experience is the person rather than something that happens to
the person (Knowles 1990). A negative self-concept in turn blocks motivation for autonomous learning (Tough 1971, 1979; Rogers 1983).

Factors influencing the process of portfolio preparation

The properties of the other five categories provided evidence of factors
which could help or hinder the process of portfolio preparation. These
influences can be divided into two main groups summarized in Table 2.3.
Some factors were logistical in that they motivated or blocked motivation

Table 2.3 Logistical and psychological factors which influenced the process of portfolio preparation and consequently development

Category	Logistical factors	Psychological factors
Reasons for doing a portfolio	Meeting requirements	Having to
		Realization of a useful purpose
Compiling content	Language writing skills	Getting it right
	Knowing what's required	Writing about self
	Collecting evidence	Objectivity versus subjectivity
	Gap in experience	
	Lack of course attendance	
Reflection		Valuing technical–rational knowledge above experience
Effect of others	Not being allowed to be innovative	Sharing problems and ideas
Time	Time-consuming	Encroachment of work on home life
Finishing		Coping with an ongoing process

as physical resources. For example, the large amount of time involved in compiling a portfolio and constraints on innovation in the clinical area, recognized by Tough (1971, 1979). Other factors acted as psychological motivators or blocks. For example, resentment at having to do a portfolio blocks readiness to learn (Knowles 1990) whilst working in a group can validate the enterprise and the degree to which experience, as opposed to technical–rational knowledge, is valued.

Discussion

The group in this study was small which restricts the drawing of inferences to the total population. It is, nevertheless, valid to draw logical inferences that reflect similar specific situations (Greenwood 1984) and to illustrate theoretical principles (Kent and Maggs 1992) as done here. My own lack of research experience also meant that this study was intended as an exploratory piece to provide direction for future work, as well as to clarify how best to help nurses with their portfolios. The findings do, however, indicate some potential for portfolios as instruments for developing reflectivity and highlights some of the factors which may help or hinder this.

Is the process of portfolio preparation in itself developmental?

The group of nurses in this project undertook preparation of their portfolios to meet the requirements of PREPP (UKCC 1990). As they came to understand its use, and relevance to them, however they changed to wanting to continue, which facilitates readiness to learn (Knowles 1990). In this sense, portfolio preparation can become a spur to action. As action research is also viewed as a spur for solving problems (Cohen and Manion 1989), involvement in the project may have motivated group members as much as the portfolio process itself.

Writing a portfolio initiated reflection to varying degrees which Schön (1987) sees as a form of experiential learning. The process of reflection indicated some development in the sense that individuals began to value their experience as learning, which is a characteristic of adult learning (Knowles 1990). Some also began facing blocks to their learning caused by limitations, such as lack of opportunities for innovation, in their clinical area, which is recognized by Tough (1971, 1979). The summarizing of experience and the narrative components of portfolios seem to be the areas which trigger this process.

Whilst reflection may raise awareness of our own lack of confidence, and the situations which have caused it, the anxiety generated by thinking about experiences which do not fit our existing constructs may be too threatening and block reflection (Mezirow 1990) and therefore learning. Mentors can help the facing of threatening experiences, through acknowledgement that problematic incidents do occur, and by showing that self-disclosure of such incidents does not result in damage to self-esteem. Working in groups with colleagues can also provide an arena for: sharing and giving feedback on problems (Kemmis 1985), confronting resistances (Heron 1989) and improving recall (Newell 1992). Colleagues can then influence the portfolio process as clarified in the category 'effect of others'.

The complexity of adult development through learning is demonstrated by Rogers (1992) whereby a cluster of activities, including awareness, education input, decision-making and action, interact simultaneously. Similarly, I found a cluster of activities and influential factors occurring in the portfolio process, causing confusion for researchers and researched. These include reflecting, writing, compiling content and listening to others. It is difficult to reflect this complexity in a report which by its nature is presented in a linear fashion.

I think that the first research question was ambitious given the constraints of time and resources. It has been far easier to identify the factors influencing the developmental process than to pin down the developmental process itself. There is an indication of the beginnings of change. Rogers (1992) suggests that ultimately the developmental goal is concerned with a process rather than a state, and an initiative which can enable the beginning of such a process should be viewed positively whilst the limitations are recognized.

If so, what are the factors influencing this developmental process?

The identified categories summarized in Table 2.3 tended to influence the portfolio process by either motivating group members to continue with the process or by blocking motivation. These factors do to some extent reflect the barriers to learning outlined by Tough (1971, 1979). Interestingly, some of the difficulties experienced were actually viewed as useful by group members. This was notably so in the case of the narrative which, although difficult to compile because it required writing about oneself, helped clarify learning from past experience: 'reflection-on-action'.

The suggested three key areas of content for a portfolio caused varying problems. The first area of summarizing experience caused less problems because it resembled writing a curriculum vitae, albeit probably in more detail than for a job application. As well as the problem with the subjective nature of a narrative (writing about self) difficulties were experienced in deciding how far back to reflect on experiences. Some group members looked back throughout their careers, which raises the questions of why they chose to do this and to what extent was it purposeful. Given that for some this resulted in learning about themselves and how they were developing, it would ultimately be something for each individual to decide. The problems reported with actual writing skills, required for these sections in particular, mirror Budnick and Beaver's (1984) own experiences. Walker (1985) also reports the confusion felt by learners trying to write reflective journals.

Collecting evidence to support learning experiences, whether course certificates or examples of initiatives undertaken in current areas of practice, was not generally a problem. Those who had not undertaken courses or who felt their practice area was resistant to innovation did, however, have difficulties with finding things to include in this section.

Overall, the three key areas used as a framework for portfolios did prove useful, although it may be simplistic to keep these three elements in separate sections. There is probably overlap between having an experience, reflecting on that experience and providing evidence of learning from the experience.

Conclusions

The choice of action research as the methodological approach has enabled the drawing together of the various strands in this project. These are: the facilitation process, the research process, reflection on my own practice and learning, and the implementation of a change initiative, albeit a small one. As a result, it has reinforced my belief in the philosophy of research, as a personal process for the researcher and the researched (for me and for the group) as well as contributing to the dialogue on portfolios within the nursing profession (for them).

It seems to me that the most valuable aspect of portfolios is the emphasis they place on experience as a learning opportunity that is at least as valuable as courses and study days. As a result, portfolio preparation may help nurses learn to value their experience as learning, through reflection, and subsequently themselves. It seems, however, that various aspects of portfolios need further thought. These are: clarification of content requirements, guidelines and criteria for assessment, particularly with regard to reregistration, and the means for continuing evaluation of their effects. Most importantly, the means by which their implementation is to be facilitated needs careful planning so that nurses can come to recognize their usefulness and view them as a positive experience.

References

Atkinson, R., Atkinson, R., Smith, E., Bem, D. and Hilgard, E. (1990) *Introduction to Psychology*, 10th edn. San Diego, CA: Harcourt Brace Jovanovich.

Barber, P. (1989) Developing the 'person' of the professional carer, in S. Hinchcliffe, S. Norman and J. Schoeber (eds) *Nursing Practice and Health Care*. Sevenoaks, Kent: Edward Arnold.

Boyd, E. M. and Fales, A. W. (1983) Reflective learning: Key to learning experience. *Journal of Humanistic Psychology*, 23(2): 99–117.

Brookfield, S. (1986) *Understanding and Facilitating Adult Learning*. Milton Keynes: Open University Press.

Budnick, D. and Beaver, S. (1984) A student perspective on the portfolio. *Nursing Outlook*, 32(5): 268–9.

Burnard, P. (1991) A method of analysing interview transcripts in qualitative research. *Nurse Education Today*, 11(6): 461–6.

Cayne, J. (1992) 'Situational analysis: The factors influencing the provision of continuing education for nurses working on an orthopaedic/trauma ward.' Unpublished work for the BEd (Hons). South Bank University, London.

Cohen, L. and Manion, L. (1989) *Research Methods in Education*, 3rd edn. London: Routledge.

DeGroot, A. (1988) Scientific inquiry in nursing: A model for a new age. *Advances in Nursing Science*, 10(3): 1–21.

Field, P. and Morse, J. (1985) *Nursing Research: The Application of Qualitative Approaches*. Beckenham, Kent: Croom Helm.

Ford, M. and Olhausen, M. (1991) 'Portfolio assessment in teacher education: Impact on students' beliefs, attitudes and habits.' Paper presented at the annual meeting of the National Reading Conference. Palm Springs, CA, December.

Gartside, G. (1990) Personal profiling. *Nursing*, 4(8): 9–11.

Glaser, B. G. and Strauss, A. (1967) *The Discovery of Grounded Theory*. Chicago, IL: Aldine.

Glen, S. and Hight, N. (1992) Portfolios: An 'affective' assessment strategy? *Nurse Education Today*, 12(6): 416–23.

Greenwood, J. (1984) Nursing research: A position paper. *Journal of Advanced Nursing*, 9(1): 77–82.

Guba, E. and Lincoln, Y. (1981) *Effective Evaluation: Improving the Usefulness of Evaluation Results Through Responsive and Naturalistic Approaches*. San Francisco, CA: Jossey-Bass.

Heron, J. (1989) *The Facilitator's Handbook*. London: Kogan Page.

Jaques, D. (1984) *Learning in Groups*. Beckenham, Kent: Croom Helm.

Jarvis, P. (1987) *Adult Learning in the Social Context*. Beckenham, Kent: Croom Helm.

Jarvis, P. (1992) Reflective practice and nursing. *Nurse Education Today*, 12(3): 174–81.

Kemmis, S. (1985) Action research and the politics of reflection, in D. Boud, R. Keogh and D. Walker (eds) *Reflection: Turning Experience into Learning*. London: Kogan Page.

Kent, J. and Maggs, C. (1992) *An Evaluation of Pre-registration Midwifery Education in England: A Research Project for the Department of Health, Working Paper 1, Research Design*. Bath: Maggs Research Associates.

Knapp, J. (1975) *A Guide to Assessing Prior Experience Through Portfolios*. Princeton, NJ: Education Testing Service, Cooperative Assessment of Experiential Learning.

Knowles, M. (1978) *Self-Directed Learning: A Guide for Learners and Teachers*. Chicago, IL: Follet.

Knowles, M. (1990) *The Adult Learner: A Neglected Species*, 4th edn. Houston, TX: Gulf Publishing.

Kolb, D. (1984) *Experiential Learning*. Englewood Cliffs, NJ: Prentice Hall.

Lambeth, S., Volden, C. and Oeschle, L. (1989) Portfolios: They work for RNs. *Journal of Nursing Education*, 28(19): 42–4.

Lewin, K. (1946) Action research and minority problems. *Journal of Social Issues*, 2.

Lyte, V. and Thompson, I. (1990) The diary as a formative teaching and learning aid incorporating means of evaluation and re-negotiation of clinical learning objectives. *Nurse Education Today*, 10(3): 228–31.

McNiff, J. (1988) *Action Research Principles and Practice*. London: Routledge.

Marsh, H. and Lasky, P. (1984) The professional portfolio: Documentation of prior learning. *Nursing Outlook*, 32(5): 264–7.

Mezirow, J. (1990) *Fostering Critical Reflection in Adulthood*. San Francisco, CA: Jossey-Bass.

Miller, M. A. (1992) 'Reflections on reflection.' Unpublished thesis for the MSc in Counselling Psychology. London: City University.

Miller, M. and Daloz, L. (1989) Assessment of prior learning: Good practices assure congruity between work and education. *Equity and Excellence*, 24(3): 30–4.

Mitchell, J. (1983) Case and situation analysis. *Sociological Review*, 31: 187–211.

Newell, R. (1992) Anxiety, accuracy and reflection: The limits of professional development. *Journal of Advanced Nursing*, 17(11): 1326–33.

Oeschle, L., Volden, C. and Lambeth, S. (1990) Portfolios and RNs: An evaluation. *Journal of Nursing Education*, 29(2): 54–9.

Porter, S. (1993) Nursing research conventions: Objectivity or obfuscation? *Journal of Advanced Nursing*, 18(1): 137–43.

Powell, J. (1989) The reflective practitioner in nursing. *Journal of Advanced Nursing*, 14(7): 824–32.

Reason, P. and Marshall, J. (1988) Research as personal process, in D. Boud (ed.) *Developing Student's Autonomy*, 2nd edn. London: Kogan Page.

Reason, P. and Rowan, P. (1981) *Human Inquiry: A Source Book of New Paradigm Research*. Chichester: John Wiley and Sons.

Rogers, A. (1992) *Adults Learning for Development*. London: Cassell

Rogers, C. (1983) *Freedom to Learn for the Eighties*. Columbus, OH: Merrill.

Schön, D. (1987) *Educating the Reflective Practitioner*. San Francisco, CA: Jossey-Bass.

Stenhouse, L. (1975) *An Introduction to Curriculum Research and Design*. London: Heinemann.

Tough, A. (1971, 1979) *The Adults Learning Projects*, 2nd edn. Ontario: Ontario Institute for Studies in Education.

United Kingdom Central Council (UKCC) (1990) *The Post Registration Education and Practice Project (PREPP)*. London: UKCC.

Walker, D. (1985) Writing and reflection, in D. Boud, R. Keogh and D. Walker (eds) *Reflection: Turning Experience into Learning*. London: Kogan Page.

Walker, E. (1992) The person professional profile. *Nursing*, 5(7): 10–11.

Webb, C. (1989) Action research: Philosophy, methods and personal experiences, *Journal of Advanced Nursing*, 14(5): 403–10.

Webb, C. (1992) The use of the first person in academic writing: Objectivity, language and gatekeeping. *Journal of Advanced Nursing*, 17(6): 747–52.

A POSTSCRIPT TO NURSING

Nicky James

Fieldwork: on a late shift, September 1981, Staff Nurse in charge of a continuing care unit

That evening I served out only the main courses, and left whoever was around to serve pudding. I gave only one person a mouthwash, instead of the normal five and practised what I was going to say when I phoned Andrea. How do you tell a 19-year-old that her father is about to die? Michael Mills, the social worker, rang and said he'd come if Andrea wanted him. She was to phone him. I thought: 'That'll muck up his Friday evening at home.' When I did get through to Andrea my words did not come out as calmly as I wanted. Without swamping her I wanted to find out if she was by herself, would she manage, how would Susie be, and how prepared was she for his death? I didn't want to frighten her, but I wanted her here quickly. I told her about Michael Mills and asked her if she wanted me to contact any of her relatives.

Life in the rest of the unit was going on like clockwork, though Fran said: 'I was so happy when I came on . . . but this place today. It's going to be a hard shift.'

I went with Anna to make Ronald Saunders look as comfortable as possible, as much for Andrea and the relatives and us as for him, then went for my break with everyone knowing that I wanted to catch Andrea for a chat before she went in to see her father. Change in appearance can be a shock.

On the 6 p.m. drug round Ethel (age 92) gave us a smile and a grouch as we fed her the medicine, which restored a sense of an ordinary day, and poor Mrs Straw, the day's new admission, was so nervous and scared she needed somebody just to sit with her for a while. But we didn't have time. Mrs Harrison refused the extra dose of diamorphine we offered her to make it easier to turn her. Retrospectively we decided that she managed her pain much better than we did, positively and usefully to make herself feel alive. We thought that we wanted her to have more medicine for our benefit not hers.

Andrea timed it beautifully and arrived as we finished the drugs. I took her to the quiet room, and left her to ring her aunt and uncle before she saw her father, intending to go in with her, but she found the new room by herself. I didn't know whether to intrude or not.

Fran passed me and said: 'Gawd Nicky, you're actually doing some work

today. But you're managing all right. Not getting upset about it.' I was
pleased that my performance did not reflect my inner disorganization.

Mr Saunders died without anyone in there, which seemed a pity. But
you can never predict the exact moment and can hang around for hours.
A friendly doctor from the adjacent hospital came over to certify him
dead, and encouraged Susan, the enrolled nurse, and me to use the
opthalmoscope to look into his eyes to see the changes that occur with
death. It was educational, and incongruous with our affection for Ronald.
I fumbled the words as I told Andrea and her aunt and uncles in the quiet
room, and asked them if they wanted to see the body. She did not, but
they did.

Anna and I laid Ronald out, while Susan filled in all the forms. I was
surprised at Anna's determined efficiency. Instead of the usual grin she
was grim and quiet. It stopped my flippancy to see how much his death
mattered to her despite the many she had seen. Tending to be guided by
whoever I was with, sometimes we behaved as if the body was still a
person to be treated with gentle attention. Other times it was an empty
shell, and comments on being withheld entry at the pearly gates because
the paper knickers were on inside out were not irreverent, because the
person had gone.

We washed him, dressed him in clean pyjamas and between us sorted
out the uncertainties of what to pack in the black plastic bag to go home
and what to throw away. Imagining the wrench of things being unpacked
the other end. You know what to do about half-used bottles of orange
squash and flannels. You chuck them. And the teddy bear lent by the
6-year-old would go back, with the cards wishing him well. But used
pyjamas and their father's well-worn razor we wanted to throw away and
knew we couldn't. I took the property to Andrea and asked her to sign for
it, which she did without opening the bag to check it. And then: 'Do you
know if you want him to be buried or cremated?' What a question to ask
within an hour of the death! But it makes a difference to the certification.
To my immense relief the question did not jar, and there was a plot next
to his father. I suspect it is easy for nurses to overestimate their importance at these times of numbness, but there is a fear that you might say
the key wrong thing and make their sorrow worse, and perhaps your own.

Taking the uncles along to the room, I asked if they thought Andrea
and Susie would manage all right, whilst thinking to myself, do I stay in
the room with them, and for how long, or just go? I stayed for moments
as they reflected on his life, and then left them. They remained only minutes longer, went back to the quiet room, and all of them left together.
The tin trunk was ordered from the porters for after the visitors had gone
at 8 p.m.

Before writing the Kardex and day report on each person's condition,
I nipped in to see everyone first. Otherwise, especially in a unit like this,
you can write that Mrs X is satisfactory, and then find that it is not so.
In the men's four-bedded room Mrs Whyte, visiting her husband, asked
what had happened to Ronald. She was upset when I told her. It was
a great temptation just to say he was very ill with the hope that she
would not ask again, but then an endless circle of evasion and half-truths
can start.

At about 8.15 the nurses had a public and unofficial tea-break at the nurses' station, in the middle of the unit. Anna had brought in apple pie for us all, and after the patients had been given the drinks they wanted, we helped ourselves. Since things had quietened down, this delightful ritual continued as usual. Susan offered to write the day report, but I said I would, and suspected myself of unreasonably asserting my status. They went back to work while I carried on writing. I hadn't finished when the three night staff arrived together, early, just after 9 p.m. for 9.15. Anna and Fran went off, leaving Susan to answer the patients' bells while I gave report. We discussed what had happened during the day and I gave details of the new lady in more depth before we talked at length about Mrs Harrison and Mrs Benedict.

By 9.45 Susan had left and I'd finished the writing. On the way off I went to say goodbye to Mr Benedict, who was in the quiet room and going to stay the night. His son was there. I was introduced and we talked of this and that and Mrs Benedict. Bill, the son, was smashing with Mr Benedict, letting his dad be proud of him and arguing with him occasionally about army stories. They seemed extraordinarily normal. Billy said to me that I must want to go home – which I did because I was tired, but I didn't know how to get away without being heartless or offensive. An awful thought was that Mrs Benedict would die soon, and I did not want to be there. You want to make each person's death as personal to the family as possible, but sometimes you run out of steam.

At 11 p.m. I left the unit to drive home, thinking I hadn't managed well, because a measure of that is that you are off on time. It was the saddest shift in eight months of fieldwork – the kind that would become folklore – and I felt wrung out.

When I got home I delivered a monologue on the day. In turn, I was told of the party of primary school kids taken round the big farm we lived on. They'd spent hours seeing the cows, feeding the bull, looking at the chickens, in the dairy, whilst draped over the adults, squealing and excited. Somehow that seemed to balance things out, a bit.

> Nicky, you're sort of like a P.S. in a letter. Not part of the main body of the nursing team, but still important.
>
>   Night nurse at the hospital

> This is our pet sociologist who's working on the unit and studying us. She's found out all sorts of interesting things.
>
>   Continuing care unit Sister, introducing me to an outsider

Narrowing down the task

Not knowing how the research system worked granted me the luxury of submitting, unperturbed, an outline, both vague and short, which managed to supply me with a department from which to work, and an initial two years' money from a central fund, with the possibility of a third year. The department was where I had done my undergraduate degree, and the mixed blessings of familiarity saved at least some of the groundwork of establishing myself. My supervisor, a vital ingredient whose importance I had not recognized, had overseen the undergraduate dissertation from which the postgraduate study was to develop. We agreed with minimal discussion to continue with each other. Approachable and non-directive as he was, he left me to discover a problem that interested me from reading which included spiritualism, psychoanalysis, census data, ethics, medicine, government reports, and so on. Somehow from this bewildering wealth, a question had to be chosen that could be followed up to reach some kind of conclusion. The distractions of philosophy held no more appeal than the abstractions of grand theory, so it was fortuitous that I was able to build on the tensions I found between being an academic and being a nurse.

Nurses *do* things as their work . . . If they are not doing something physical they are not working, and to be in a sociology department concentrating on the written word and discussion seemed egocentric and indulgent. Thus one of the easiest decisions on how to solidify the nebulous thesis was to make it empirical, using previous knowledge. Such a decision had a huge impact, far from clear at the time, because it not only structured the projected three years into a manageable timetable, but to me implied a particular way of thinking, which excluded number crunching and hypothesis testing – both, then, sociology of derision. Thinking in terms of interpersonal relations, I wanted to know how people affected each other in looking after the dying (which at the time I took to be a passive event for the patient) and where the power of decision lay.

Intertwined with considering more specifically what I wanted to do was the input from others. During the initial weeks I discovered there were different groups of people relevant to the project – outsiders, university staff, other postgraduates and friends. Needless to say, these shifted categories over time. I also worked on the basis that there were two types of problems, acceptable ones you feel you can ask about and unacceptable ones which are more difficult to ask and which are matched more carefully against the audience.

The staff, whom I already knew, although unclear on the resources available for postgraduates . . . were a source of endless suggestions of people to see and expansive lists of books and articles to read. Knowing that they could not all be seen or read, it was difficult to evaluate which to choose. To optimize their proffered help required knowing what I was doing at the very time I was least sure.

The list of references grew alarmingly in inverse proportion to the clarity of the problem. Some friends were intrigued enough to be useful sounding boards, asking questions which, in encouraging me to explain simply, helped sort the irrelevant from the necessary to the enlightening. Others were part of the network keeping me informed of radio and television programmes, talks and newspaper articles, also providing light entertainment when the dark side of death was looming large.

In January, four months after starting, I attended a multidisciplinary terminal care course with nurses, social workers, clergy and a few doctors. From taking embarrassingly more notes than anyone else, and feeling like neither nurse nor researcher, it occurred to me that spoken repetition on the course of written phrases in the literature, which encapsulate 'good' terminal care, such as 'teamwork', 'individual patient assessment', 'death with dignity', could be used as categories of observation. Sociologically this carried all the dangers of using language generated within and by the groups being observed, but they were of value because commendable as ideals, though I thought there might be some obstacles to their practice. They also served the useful function of giving credibility to a study within the medical settings in which I thought it might be pertinent to work.

A few weeks later when 'The role of the nurse in the care of the dying' had been achieved as the working title, I began to formulate the kind of fieldwork I was going to do, and devise ways of becoming acceptable to nursing administrators – hoping to use the sway of past nursing training. So 'staff' spread from academics to National Health administrators.

Despite the profoundly good advice of an anthropologist who told me that projects should be limited to take home life into account, it took a formal discussion with three nursing hierarchs to alter my grandiose schemes. The meeting was a fascinating struggle between my two roles of nurse and researcher, with the former winning. Although medical sociology was well established locally, I had thought that being introduced so officially to people I wanted to work with on the wards might make me a threat. Instead, using old nursing contacts, I made my own way.

In the proposal to the nursing administrators, submitted before I went to see them, I tried to 'sell' myself by predicting what they would like, and also what they would dislike, so that it could be counteracted. The proposal was deliberately left flexible so that there was room for manoeuvre, but my main doubt was that they would tolerate an observer. Why should they? To try to overcome that, I made a commitment to working free, instead of being an onlooker, and the more I thought about it the more I thought it would provoke interesting data . . .

As it was I totally misjudged their reading of the proposal. Instead of being flexible it looked as though I did not know what I was doing, and though they welcomed nursing research, there was some anxiety over someone who wanted to be integrated. The effectiveness that the authority of nursing administrators can have on those they train showed, and I acquiesced to their suggestions that I drop totally the community part of a scheme which had included time to be spent in a community, in a hospital, and in a hospice.

In the report on the meeting I noted that 'I went in optimistic and came out feeling like a grilled sardine – small, squashed and hot'.

Having given me their tentative support, the administrators continued to meet me intermittently, and they helped devise the proposal to go before the Ethical Committee. At the time it caused enormous concern since the project could be stopped, but once it was accepted the whole thing vanished as unimportant, with the exception that they made me have a nurse supervisor. A senior tutor at the Infirmary Nursing School, she not only let me talk at her, but eased my way into the nursing school, allowing me freely to use the library and video facilities, and by the end setting up interviews with other nursing tutors and a forum for discussion of what I was doing. It was part of my integration back into the nursing establishment.

Not until the end of the first year with a methodology summer school, did the relief and revelation come that other postgraduates had trouble with their filing systems, how to take notes, and how to distinguish fact from opinion in their own writing, let alone other people's. I found that everyone struggled to write, or avoid it, that their theoretical base was not the clear shining light illuminating their path that I assumed it should be. Indeed other participant observers, like me, were at a loss to know how data fits theory or theory fits data. That these were not necessarily difficulties solved as an undergraduate indicated that some of the questions I had thought to be too obvious to ask about were part of learning research. Others too suffered from degrees of lack of professional confidence that I had not formerly thought commensurate with the status of a postgraduate, and as we chatted over the minutiae of our research problems, informally as much as in guided sessions, so our academic contacts grew to good effect and came to be renewed at future conferences. I found this invaluable.

A one-month hospice course during the first year had firmed up my supposition that there was a gap between the rhetoric of 'good' terminal care, and what happens when it is practised, and also indicated some of the future problems of participant observation. As the time for the bulk of the fieldwork was approaching, I anticipated difficulties in writing at the end of a shift. I therefore devised a limited number of A4 forms (to allow for later adaptation) – partly numbers and cases, and partly descriptive – to ease the way into getting the shift into some kind of perspective. To this were to be added tape-recordings of what the shift had felt like, although it was only once the fieldwork was underway that sheets of 'odd thoughts' developed. They made no attempt to be a coherent part of the data, but just seemed brilliantly insightful at the time.

Another aspect of preparation was to introduce myself and the study to the hospital ward and the continuing care unit where I was to work – ostensibly to ask their permission, although I felt they had little choice once the doctors and the Ethical Committee had agreed to it.

The sister on the medical ward which was used mainly for heart patients was exceptionally open-minded, forward thinking and relaxed, but saw little point in having a researcher into dying on the ward when there were not that many deaths – which was difficult when the numbers of deaths apparently went up when I was there. The common quip about me being a Jonah had something of an edge to it. In contrast, the sister on the continuing care unit, a place known as something of a deathhouse, was anxious to present the staff and patients as a happy and unified family – which I did not believe, but had qualms at the prospect of exposing. In both places I sat in on the report when all the nurses on duty regularly gather together, to explain what I wanted to do, neither wanting to appear an academic know-all nor to make them feel like the objects of study. (In the end, one of the ways I was accepted was to be thought of as clever – only clever people are at university – but a bit dim at practical things.) I could only explain in general terms what I intended to do, pointing out that the outcome of the research was unclear – it was exactly why I was going to do the study – and so like many researchers, deliberately or not, I failed to convey what the research was about.

To maintain my identity as a researcher, what I wore to work (it was noticeable that I used 'work' to describe nursing but rarely to describe writing or university events) became of symbolic significance. I was in a quandary, as I did not want to deliberately obscure my identity to pretend I was not doing research, but also wanted to be accepted as one of the team, though the administrators wanted me to be visibly different. The white coat was discarded in favour of a nursing dress, but I was not to have a hat or epaulettes which denote the stage and type of training. As was intended these careful omissions generated an awareness of my difference, but by the end of fieldwork in the hospital, before I started in the unit, I had acquired both. Usually reluctant to wear uniforms, not feeling I belonged was disquieting and I made the effort to be allowed the privilege of wearing a white paper hat, and the pink epaulettes of a staff nurse. Going native.

Which is the right information?

The great day came. The proper start of fieldwork. On for an early shift, I got up at 5.30 a.m. after a terrible night's sleep, drove with jumbled thoughts to the hospital, changed in the sisters' locker room (a measure of my confusing status to administrators as well as to myself), and went down early to the ward where my name had been added to the nursing rota. (Despite my being on the rota, no nurse was to be displaced as the result of my being there. It would have caused union problems as I was unpaid. It was also to my advantage because most nurses are reluctant to be 'lent' when there are too many nurses on the ward, and it could have created bad feeling.) The shift was a daunting muddle to me. We had report and unlike the others, I was not allocated to work with someone but left to find my own jobs. The Sister thought she was being helpful, but I felt lost. A few remarks from my fieldnotes:

> I didn't know what I was doing, and the lack of routine was very undermining, or rather the lack of knowledge of the routine was very undermining to me. I felt that I had no independence on the ward because I nearly always had to ask people if I wanted to do, or thought I ought to do, something.

> One of the problems all during today has been the vast input of possible information, and not knowing how to select it. I'd already decided that for the first couple of days I'd concentrate on my own socialization, the acquiring of the routine, learning about the ward and so on to be able to write down the timetable of the nursing day, but even so.

Confusion and doubt is part of any nurse's move to a new ward, but I had forgotten that and I found it difficult to make sense of things as a nurse, let alone a researcher. Even as I settled down to doing auxiliary-nurse-type of work, though still having coffee in Sister's office, I was casting about for what it was that I was trying to discover. Good social scientists manage to establish valuable facts. My observations seemed to lack that authority. And field researchers always live, to some extent, with the disquieting notion that they are gathering the wrong data, that they should be observing or asking questions about another event or practice, instead of the present one.

Truth, objectivity and bias loomed large in my thinking throughout the fieldwork, and increasingly quantitative research seemed to hold the enticing allure of being 'scientific'. It was not until I was well back out of the nursing that what had been written during it looked as though it had any purpose or explanatory use.

It was intended that the research would generate its own emphases, but I had needed not only a product to sell to the people whose aid I wanted to enlist, but also to give some direction to my thinking – as for instance in the forms I made.

In submitting the proposal to the nursing administrators I had made a mental note to beware that I did not get taken in by my own propaganda, to remember that my interest was skewed to people who were thought to be ill and people who helped look after them, rather than patients and nurses, that I was being a nurse merely as a means to research. Once involved, that seemed heartlessly instrumental. When they went to supper, work stopped for them, as they assumed it did for me, and their trust, which I wanted, was discomforting. Occasionally passing outrageous remarks to make it clear that I was not one of them, giving them a chance to defend themselves against me, did little but salve my conscience. However, as they were subjects of study to me, so to some extent was I subject to study and use by them. In attempting to keep free enough from the restrictions of hypotheses to let the data indicate the important issues, so I was open to be buffeted by the most powerful influences and friendships. The result is that the majority of quotable quotes came from few people, and my preoccupations were those of the places and people with whom I worked. A useful bias.

. . .

Unanticipated and useful additions to my knowledge were also made as my status changed on the hospital ward, but more obviously so in the continuing care unit. In both places I tried to fit in by doing what was asked of me, but not taking leading decisions, and I had thought that I would work in the background with the auxiliaries. Not only do the auxiliaries not stay in the background, but I was known to be a staff nurse. By the fourth day in the hospital, when I asked a student nurse about doing something, she said: 'You decide, you're in charge.' When time was short and the drug round was due, I was qualified to do it, and to take charge of the drug keys when other trained staff were off the ward. Adopting different roles in the hierarchy is what everyone but the most senior do every day, and that on one shift I could be in charge of the continuing care unit and the next be cleaning the sluice – auxiliary territory – pointed up just how conscious and specific the hierarchies are . . .

As my time at the hospital came to a close, I decided that a longer and perhaps more reflective discussion on the nurses' thoughts about their

work would be a helpful addition to the remarks and brief debates that
I heard as they organized and cared for the patients. On night duty there
had been more opportunity to talk casually and at length, but on days it
needed to be arranged beforehand. I went to Betty's house as researcher
and workmate, but after a five-hour rambling conversation which included her husband and child, interspersed with lunch and afternoon tea,
the difficulty of remembering what had been said made leaving a tape-
recorder running an attractive proposition. I asked the Sister if she minded
me having one there as she and I talked round a few subjects, and she was
relaxed enough to ignore it. I did not do enough taping at the hospital
before I left to take account of the kind of effect I was having.

During a two-month break from nursing for a reappraisal of where I'd
got so far, I gave a seminar paper in the department which, though not
obvious then, became one of the main outlines for the final thesis. This,
together with the regular meetings with my supervisor throughout the
fieldwork, allowed some of my thoughts on terminal care nursing to
coalesce. When I went to work on the purpose-built continuing care unit
I hoped, somewhat deviously, that getting people to talk about their
thoughts on how care of the dying should be approached would give a
helpful comparison with what could be observed of their practice of it. I
postponed doing this until I was better known, but when an excellent
nurse was about to leave, I was provoked to start. People knew me and my
ideas too well for me to be able to interview them, and although there
were four general areas I wanted to ask about, having a 'conversation' was
more appropriate. Taping saved intrusive scribbling. I anticipated that
everyone worked with me and teased me well enough for the conversations not to bother them too much. They were either at people's houses
or at the unit, whichever they preferred, but the variations in how easy
people found it, and their fluency in the more formal talk, were enormous. Until I listened to the tapes retrospectively, I did not realize the
resistance, despite familiarity, of the power structure between interviewer
and informant. In some cases I got the power balances quite wrong even
when I had learnt to sit through the silences, though in others they
organized themselves to make it easier. I arrived at Mary's to find that she
had invited Jessica round so they could do it together, and we all had
lovely afternoon tea. This in itself was good data, not to be missed out
and whilst it was part of the 'gossamer of ideas' on how nurses control
their circumstances, I was constantly concerned as to its validity (to whom?)
and acceptability (to whom?) as social science, prompted by what I thought
to be its unacceptability within medical circles. They obviously talked
over the conversations with each other as they happened, and inevitably
the discussions gave pause for reflection – I was told so several times – but
how they affected behaviour was impossible to detect.

The unit was something of a showcase, built as it was with money from
the local community and with the purpose of providing care for cancer
patients. The Sister in charge was therefore more involved than most in
showing visitors round, thereby, with some anxiety, putting herself on
show. She looked after me as thoughtfully as she looked after the others,
giving me time in the quiet room to write up notes, and I suspect she was
both pleased and somewhat disquieted to have me there. Although we

were both careful in our management of it, it is possible that I may have been a threat to her, and as far as I can remember, despite being there for five months, I did not publicly air my views in front of her as vehemently as I did in other chatting groups. Mutual support is an important contribution to maintaining a happy atmosphere in terminal care units, feared and criticized as they often are by outsiders, and stressful within. My criticisms, through regular discussion and deliberate distancing, were more succinct than most, and it was something of a dilemma when asked my opinion.

A dysfunction built into the research, for which I had made inadequate provision, was the constant prodding at the defence mechanisms which are a means of continuing at the unit. If I pushed the others too far they would evade, avoid or tell me to shut up, but my own defences were also under scrutiny and the more I was perturbed by exposing them, the more my reluctance to write up at the end of the day grew. I was enjoying the nursing. For the research, philosophy, the structure of the National Health Service, and numbers became easier lines of thought. None of them had anything to do with people . . .

TALKING TO PEOPLE AND ASKING QUESTIONS

Introduction

The four chapters in this section are about gathering data by asking people questions, as opposed to working with them and seeing how things are done – participant observation – as illustrated in the last section. The papers differ along a continuum of structure. In the first, very little pre-conception is imposed on the topic, and the method of interviewing is generally described as *open* or *ethnographic*. Women are asked about their lives and experiences and encouraged to talk about themselves and their histories in their own terms; there is a research agenda, but the researchers make every effort not to let it alter what the informants want to say about themselves. (A fair amount of this kind of interviewing, and less formal 'chats', goes on in participant observation research as well, as you will have realized from Kirkham's and James's chapters in Section A.)

The crucial stage of research is the beginning, when the important decisions are taken which will affect what can be concluded from our work. The second paper in this section describes the planning stage of a piece of survey research into Plymouth's heart patients and the consequences of the trip to London some of them have to make for treatment; the research aims to provide understanding of how much this trip disrupts their and their families' lives and to gather information which can be used to improve services to such patients. It outlines some of the decisions that had to be made and some of the alternative approaches which had to be discarded. It demonstrates how sampling is worked out in a real-life situation and how groups are selected for comparison, to maximize the 'pay-off' from the data. It also raises some of the ethical and political issues which researchers face at the design stage.

Chapter 6 describes survey research into home helps and district nurses and the work they do for older clients. The idea of a survey is that all the respondents are asked the same structured questions in the same way – presented with a constant 'stimulus' – so that differences between their answers are due to differences in their character or experience, not differences in the way the information was collected. (We talk about surveys as ways of asking structured questions, but the same principles hold for surveys in which the researcher systematically observes what is going on in, for example, different school playgrounds or different magistrates' courts or different casualty departments; survey data do not have to be verbal.) Chapter 6 is an overview of the work, giving headline results from questionnaires to clients and to the home helps and district nurses. Chapter 7 focuses on one aspect, a questionnaire sent to district nurses and home helps in which they were asked who should do which tasks in a series of fictional cases or *vignettes*. This is a technique which is very useful for examining practice in a non-intrusive way; it is more naturalistic than just asking about policies in the abstract, but capable of more systematic variation and control than straightforward observation of whatever cases happen to occur during a period in the field.

The strengths of Chapters 6 and 7 – and of structured surveys in general – are that we have precisely comparable data for all informants, neatly categorized to facilitate comparison. Their weakness is that the data are categorized in terms of the researchers' conception of the topic area, which is not necessarily the same as the informants'. This makes them descriptively quite useful, and good tools for testing researchers' hypotheses that specified groups will answer preset questions in predictably different ways – to test theory, in other words – but not necessarily very apt for exploration and theory-building. The open interviewing technique used in Chapter 4 is better adapted to exploring how the informants see their worlds in their own terms, but the price paid for this richness of data is that it may be more difficult to compare across cases.

The difference between Chapter 4 and Chapters 6 and 7 reflects a traditional divide in discussions about research methods between 'qualitative' and 'quantitative' work. The former, exemplified by 'Leaving it to mum', owes a primary commitment to naturalism and holism. That is, it aims to be able to generalize directly from the research situation to the informants' everyday lives by imposing as little structure as possible on the situation and concentrating in the first instance in letting the informants' own voices be heard. The latter, exemplified by Chapters 6 and 7, owes a primary commitment to reliable and generalizable description and/ or the testing of hypotheses. The difference in naturalism is one of degree, not of kind, in these papers. The research on community care in Cornwall, for instance, tries to ask its questions in language that is natural for the informants, as if a naturalistic conversation were taking place. On the other hand, open interviewing is not unstructured, any more than any conversation is unstructured. Indeed, detailed analysis of open interviews reveals a degree of structure which would not be natural for an everyday conversation, with the researcher contributing far less information to the conversation than would be normal but taking far greater charge of it in the sense of determining when the subject is to be changed and when a topic needs further elaboration. The difference in holism is perhaps more than a matter of degree, however; the 'open interviewing' paper tries to set the research topic in the context of the whole lives of the participants, while Chapters 6 and 7 have predetermined areas of enquiry with which they are designed to deal in predetermined ways and using predetermined questions exploring aspects which are thought to be relevant.

Differences in approach are to some extent independent of method, however, as is demonstrated by the way the different papers approach the cluster of attitudes/beliefs/opinions. How you measure or collect these depends on how you conceptualize them. If you think of an attitude or a belief as something factual – something the person has, is aware of and can report – then the simplest thing is to ask direct questions: 'Are you satisfied with the service you have received?' or 'Who should provide the service in this case?' Alternatively, however, you could undertake open interviewing from this stance, with the same intention of taking what people said about their lives as a factual and authoritative report, true because they say it is true. If you think of attitudes as something which people have but of which they are not necessarily aware – implicit ways of judging the world or tendencies to behave in certain ways – then you might use a more indirect approach (such as, 'What do you think your job should be called?'), trying to uncover what lies *underneath* the explicit judgements that people make. Alternatively, you might undertake open interviewing, but with the intention of interpreting what was said rather than taking it at face value. If you believe that attitudes are something that people *do* – ways in which they make sense to themselves of their actions and their experiences – then you would be most likely to undertake open interviewing, to see how they form and express opinions in context-specific ways. You might, however, use either of the other approaches, but be inclined to interpret the results more cautiously and reflexively than if you held one of the other positions.

In one respect, then, the papers in this section differ in the degree of structure which they exhibit. In another, however, they are all fairly structured; the nature of the informants is carefully managed to suit the 'argument' of the research. Chapter 5 sets out to explore the experience of heart patients who travel for surgery, and their attitudes and experiences are to be illuminated by comparison with another group of patients who do not have to travel for their treatment. Chapters 6 and 7 set out to cover all interested parties – health visitors, district nurses, their organizers, their clients and the clients' informal helpers – and so the informants are selected to fall into and be representative of these groups. The points are made, again, by a series of comparisons, between district nurses and home helps. Chapter 4, though the most 'qualitative' of the papers, has the greatest degree of structuring in terms of its samples. Being concerned with the experiences of mothers of children with learning difficulties, the researchers naturally seek out a sample of such mothers. Being aware, however, that you cannot say what is specific to such mothers unless you can show differences from other kinds of mother, the researchers make an effort to find a group of mothers whose children are not labelled in this way, to act as a comparison. Although we think of qualitative research as unstructured, this kind of theoretical sampling to explore the extent to which the results are correctly understood is entirely typical both of open interviewing research and of participant observation. Comparison and contrast lie at the centre of our understanding of data; we do not understand our results until we know precisely to whom they do or do not apply.

One would traditionally expect survey reports to exhibit a fair amount of care over demonstrating that their samples are typical of the population which they purport to represent. Broadly speaking, there are five methods of assuring representation in the selection of respondents.

1 The easiest way is of course not to sample at all but to try to approach everyone, as in the Census, and this is the approach taken in Chapters 6 and 7 for the district nurse and home help questionnaires; they were sent to every member of staff.

2 Given that sampling is necessary, the best method is random sampling, where a list of the population is prepared and cases are chosen from it randomly until the desired size of sample is obtained. There can be no conscious bias in such sampling because the researcher does not control who is chosen. If the sample is reasonably large there should also be little chance of drawing a set which differs dramatically from the population in *any* respect (and, if the sampling is random, the likelihood of doing so can be estimated).

3 If random sampling is not possible, perhaps because it is not possible to list the entire sample, then different methods must be used. Researching hospital visiting, for example, we might try to sample every case arriving during a given time period, trying to pick the time period to be as typical as possible of 'normal' visiting. Under other circumstances we might sample an unknown population by taking geographical clusters (streets, houses, postcodes) and using these as the contact-points for our sample. Again we would have to ensure that we had a good spread of contact-points and were not, for example, biased towards middle-class or working-class areas. Properly done, this kind of sampling can produce something which imitates a random sampling method quite well, but inevitably with a higher chance of obtaining a biased (unrepresentative) sample.

4 Where even this is not possible, perhaps for reasons of cost, researchers will sometimes set up what is known as a quota sample design. Here you pick important variables whose population distribution is known (e.g. gender, age, class), work out how many people there ought to be in each 'cell' of the design if the sample is to resemble the population (e.g. how many young middle-class males, young middle-class females, middle-aged middle-class males, etc.) and send interviewers out to obtain that number of responses, setting no other constraint on how they find the respondents. This method is widely used in market research and also in political opinion research, where it is said to work quite well. You can imagine, however, that it is open to introducing very great biases, because interviewers are free to go for the respondents who are easiest to find at the time when they are looking, and these may not be typical of the population as a whole.

5 The worst sampling design of all is exhibited by studies which just stop people in the street, or go from house to house on a particular day, or uses some group who just have to be available (such as a class of students). It is overwhelmingly likely that these will not form a representative sample. Sometimes this is the only kind of sample available, however, as in the Cayne research about which you read in Chapter 2.

In evaluating the generalizability of research conclusions you always have to consider the quality of the sampling design, and also how representative or typical the sample actually *achieved* is likely to be. It is a very common problem of postal and other 'self-completion' surveys, for example, that response rates of less than 50 per cent are not at all uncommon and we do not necessarily know that the 50 per cent who replied are a random subset of all those who *might* have replied.

We should distinguish, however, between representative sampling and the achievement of a *typical* group. Chapter 4, for example, tries to find a typical group in the sense that every effort is made to cover a range of 'types' and circumstances, and it may well succeed in doing so, but there is no good reason to suppose that these few informants constitute a group which reflects exactly the social and personal characteristics of the population of mothers of children with learning difficulties. It is a good sample for generating description and theory, but to determine relative frequencies of characteristics in the population a different kind of research would be needed.

FOUR

LEAVING IT TO MUM: 'COMMUNITY CARE' FOR MENTALLY HANDICAPPED CHILDREN

Pamela Abbott and Roger Sapsford

The policy of 'community care' for mentally handicapped children has non-financial costs for families: work which in institutions would be wage-labour becomes unpaid work for 'Mum' when the burden of care is transferred to the family. This chapter looks at the nature and extent of such work and at the extent to which it alters the nature of the mother's life. We look also at the price which is paid by the whole family for the fact of having a mentally handicapped member – a price made up of shattered expectations which have to be rebuilt, the disturbance to family life, the reactions of others, the constraints on the mother's life, and the disturbance of normal expectations for the family's future. (The 'price' differs markedly from family to family, depending at least in part on the degree of handicap, the extent of associated physical handicaps and the social and economic situation of the family; what follows is a composite, not necessarily true to the experience of any one mother.)

The data come from two main sources. One is research which we carried out jointly during 1981 and 1982 in and around a new city in the English midlands, interviewing mothers of mentally handicapped children (and sometimes other family members who happened to be present). Sixteen families were contacted from a list extracted for us from the school rolls of two Special Schools in the new city (one designated for the mildly handicapped and one for the severely). We carried out two interviews with each mother separated by about a year, not using a formal questionnaire but rather trying for the atmosphere of a friendly chat about life and work between neighbours. Although the interviews were tape-recorded, it seemed to us that this atmosphere was readily attained in most cases – the more so because Abbott was very evidently pregnant during the early interviews. This was one main source of our information. The other source was a similar series of interviews carried out earlier by Abbott with families in an outer London suburb, contacted through the good offices of the local branch of the National Society for Mental Handicap. Although we cannot claim that either of these small-scale studies has a sample statistically representative of the population of mentally handicapped children, we would claim that together they cover a large part of the range – from the mildest of borderline handicaps to the very severe, and from pre-school children to (in Abbott's study) 'children' in their 40s. These data are contrasted with a parallel series of interviews with mothers of children who have *not* been labelled as mentally handicapped.

Reactions to handicap

One major set of costs to the family of the mentally handicapped child is the reactions which the family will have and will encounter to the fact that their child is handicapped. The family has to come to terms with altered expectations for the child, an altered perspective for the future, and the cultural stigma which attaches to the label. A family 'lifestyle' has to be built which can cope with the situation – and revised, and re-revised as time goes on. Finally, the family has to negotiate its position *vis-à-vis* the outside world and to deal with the real, expected or imagined reactions of others. This section looks at the price the family pays for its 'abnormal' member and at how family members cope with it.

The initial reaction may vary from grief to outright emotional rejection. On the one hand grief may be immediate and temporarily overwhelming:

> [The doctor] was rather brutal. I mean true enough one has to learn . . . but I left that surgery in tears . . . and I walked and I was crying as I walked along.
>
> (Mrs Neade)

Grief may be delayed but no less powerful when it does come: two of the 16 mothers to whom we spoke described long periods (in one case two or three years) of numbness, followed by some kind of breakdown. For others again there may be a period during which the child is effectively rejected:

> For about a month after I found out I didn't have any feeling for her any way – she wasn't my baby, she was just *a* baby that had got to be looked after and fed and kept clean. I couldn't pick her up and cuddle her or nothing . . . And I walked past the pram one day and she looked up at me and she smiled at me . . . she just smiled . . . after that I was all right.
>
> (Mrs Miller)

Immediate expectations are broken, and there may be disappointment and jealousy:

> Four girls, five girls who I went to school with . . . all had beautiful bouncing babies, and there was me with my poor little thing. I was a bit resentful.
>
> (Mrs Miller)

> I was most disappointed, because I thought I was going to have a beautiful-looking baby, you know. Well, she was all colours, she was bleeding all over.
>
> (Mrs King)

Immediate decisions have to be taken: to take the child home or to leave 'it' in the hospital, to seek or not to seek institutionalization after the child has gone home, to take all the small decisions which may appear to happen automatically – 'It's just part of something that happens and you just get on with it . . . you don't think about each day, do you?' – but which amount to a commitment to care in the community. The beginnings of a stance towards the outside world have also to be adopted: for example, the decision not to attempt concealment:

> the sooner people knew, I thought, the nicer for them, because there's nothing worse than looking in a pram and it's a friend, and thinking, 'Oh goodness, what can I say?'
>
> (Mrs Rushden)

Thus the first thing that has to be done by the family is to come to terms with broken expectations and altered circumstances – to do the hard work of building the beginnings of the new and different life. At this time there may also have to be a reassessment of self. Whether or not the feeling is judged irrational, there may be a denigration of self – 'I felt inadequate, I felt it must be me' (Mrs Miller) – and a need to construct some answer to the question 'Why me?' Seven of our 16 mothers mentioned some kind of 'hereditary taint' as something for which one or the other side of the family needed to take some blame – a survival in popular consciousness of the outdated science of the Eugenics Movement – and three others denied a belief in heredity with enough vehemence that one suspects the question had been an issue for the family. Fathers also may have to come to terms with 'being the sort of person' who has produced a mentally handicapped child – self-labelling can run all the more rampant because this is an area of life where it is difficult for spouses even to talk to each other, let alone talk to others outside the family – and siblings may worry about themselves and have their worries reinforced by their school friends.

All of the mothers in our new city sample had made some kind of initial working adjustment, but the same was not true of all of their husbands. Three of the 16 marriages broke up after the birth of the handicapped child – not solely because of the child's handicap, but at least in part because the husband could not accept it – and in another case the marriage was put under great strain. Most of the husbands of the women we have interviewed are described by their wives as having difficulty in coming to terms with themselves and their children, and in general it is found that stress similar in degree to the mothers but different in kind (less self-punitive, on the whole) may be detected in most fathers of mentally handicapped children (Cummings 1976). Husbands sometimes have to change their lifestyle radically in order to facilitate the adjustment of the family. Sometimes the husband's job or career has to be modified; for example, one man in our new city sample gave up several chances of promotion to save moving to another area, and another took on a fish and chip shop, with his wife, in order to be more available to the family. Substantial reorganization of normally expected roles may be necessary to preserve an otherwise normal family life; siblings may have to take on a parental role with respect to the handicapped child, and the husband may have to play more of a part in family life than is the norm.

The literature suggests that on the whole fathers become more involved in child care than those whose children are not mentally handicapped. In a survey carried out by Hunter (1980), for example, 25 per cent of employed fathers of mentally handicapped children were 'on nights' or on shift work, and therefore available to take children to clinics and in general to look after them during the day; some fathers had changed to shift work precisely for this reason. On the other hand, some studies find the opposite; Gallagher *et al.* (1983), for example, note that 'the father often plays a limited role in these families even when present'. Both in our new city sample and in the earlier South London work the predomin-ant experience was nearer to the latter state than the former – fathers did help with children, but in general no more so than might be found in some other families. The immediate stress of handicap is in any case less for employed fathers than for non-working mothers because they escape from home for substantial periods of the day. The relationship between husband and wife may well deteriorate nonetheless, as we have seen.

Thus one major 'price' which the parents of mentally handicapped children have to pay for their children is a reorganization of how the family sees itself and how life is lived within it and in interaction with others around it. A second, related price is paid in terms of the nature of the family's identity *vis-à-vis* the outside world and the consequent reac-tions of others. Mental handicap is a stigmatizing condition in our cul-ture, and it is not only the retarded themselves who carry the stigma, but also their families. Goffman (1963) refers to the sharing of another's spoilt identity as 'bearing a courtesy stigma' – the family members have a spoilt identity because of their close affiliation to someone who bears the prim-ary signs. Birenbaum (1970) suggests that the families of the mentally subnormal tend to provide a very good example of a group of people who carry this kind of courtesy stigma but who seek to maintain a normal appearance by carrying on with the 'normal' life pattern. In order to do this they maintain a 'normal' family life, avoid stigmatizing situations and retain social relationships. Sometimes this may mean a dramatic change in the nature of the social relations which are retained. The South London sample, for instance, were all active members of their local association and tended to use it as a basis for the family's social life. This was much less common among our later new city sample – the local association was far less active there – but many of the mothers at least were actively involved with the teachers and social workers of the ESN(S) school or with the newly formed parents' association at the ESN(M) school. Several mothers were also active in charitable work for the mentally handicapped – Mrs Neade, for example, had until recently been a local organizer for Home Farm Trust's fund-raising activities, and Mrs Rushden was involved in so many things that she described mental handicap as her hobby. While some were well integrated in villages or urban communities, and others in a state of 'normal' urban isolation, others tended to shape their friendships around their retarded children. In Mrs Ovenden's words,

I miss my friends. Nearly all my friends now are mothers who have children with difficulties, from the [ESN(M)] school, and they've been a great help. But some of the others! One woman kept trying to put

Clive down by getting her own child [the same age] to show him how to do things. He doesn't worry, of course, but I mind ...

In any case the problem of integration tends to become greater as the child reaches adulthood and it becomes increasingly difficult to retain an appearance of normality.

The experiences of the 11 families interviewed in the South London study varied considerably. Some felt intensely that they were stigmatized as a consequence of having a handicapped member and that other people openly displayed negative reactions towards them. These negative reactions might be displayed by relatives, friends, the 'general public' and professionals alike. Conversely others felt that everyone had been very helpful and kind. Abbott's own impressions – from looks, inflections in the voice and other cues as well as from what people said – were that they had all had disturbing experiences and that they all felt that other people regarded them as 'different', pitied them and to some extent avoided them. Also they all seemed to structure their lives as families so as to avoid possibly embarrassing situations – for example, by not asking friends to babysit, by not inviting friends or relatives to call whom they felt would be embarrassed by the presence of the subnormal member. What came over most clearly was a feeling that people's attitudes were ambivalent; that at an abstract level they experienced sympathy but that when confronted with the possibility of direct contact with the mentally handicapped they tried to avoid it. Out new city data would admit of a similar analysis.

One has to remember that the majority of people have no first-hand knowledge of the mentally handicapped. They have stereotyped images, often influenced by outdated 'scientific' knowledge and occasionally stirred up by sensationalized newspaper articles. (Attitudes towards sex and the mentally handicapped, discussed below, are a good example of this tendency.) These images more often refer to the severely than to the mildly subnormal. Shearer (1972: 3), for example, has suggested that

> it is still widely believed that mentally handicapped people are un-controlled and perverted in their sexual appetites. In the past this belief has been one of the main incentives for shutting them away in segregated institutions.

and Greengross (1976: 94) that

> the fearful myth that the mentally sick and subnormal ... are promiscuous and have voracious sexual appetites which they are incapable of satisfying responsibly or within a socially acceptable pattern of behaviour is one that still holds water for many, and although statistics keep pouring out to explode the myth, old prejudices and fears die hard.

This would seem to be a good example of how arguments developed by the Eugenics Movement and others to justify the permanent segregation of mentally handicapped people have filtered through and still influence people's perceptions of the mentally handicapped. The 'outdated' views referred to in the above quotations were clearly expressed in books and articles on the mentally subnormal in the first two decades of this century. However, the view that at least some mentally subnormal men and women have abnormal appetites is still openly stated by 'experts'. Tredgold and Soddy's influential textbook (1970) for the medical profession argued as recently as 1970 that in the case of subnormal men

> open masturbation in the presence of others, indecent exposure, indecent assault especially on immature girls, occasional rape and sexual murder are possible.
>
> (p. 90)

while in the case of

> subnormal girls . . . in some ways the problems . . . are even more intractable . . . Some subnormal girls have comparatively strong direct sex drives . . . The gratification aspects of their sexuality will be uppermost. Some girls will discover how to use their bodies to give them power over men and drift into prostitution. . . . The self-gratification aspects of their need can also drive girls into sexual promiscuity.
>
> (p. 91)

(There is indeed some evidence that mentally handicapped men commit more than their fair share of sexual offences, and that although they are not very often violent their victims are often young children. However, the total numbers of mentally handicapped men charged and convicted of such offences are very small – see Walker and McCabe, 1973.)

While scientific and social developments in the twentieth century have resulted in changes in the way the mentally handicapped are conceptualized and in methods of handling, nonetheless the beliefs of the Eugenics Movement live on to a large extent in 'popular consciousness'. The prevalence and power of the stereotype is well illustrated by a study described by one of us (Abbott 1982) of a village's reactions to the establishment of a hostel for mentally handicapped women. While many of the villagers objected vociferously to the hostel and expressed fears for the safety of the village's children, what was most revealing was the ambivalent attitudes of a group who became 'Friends of the Hostel' and visited the girls regularly. Even these women had doubts about whether the hostel should have been opened in their village and in fact shared many of the fears that they claimed were voiced by those opposed to the hostel – fears of violent and sexually uncontrolled behaviour. Similar attitudes and prejudices emerged in group dicussions which Abbott ran with full-time students in a college of further education, a generation on from the 'Friends of the Hostel' and a group selected as of sufficient academic ability to cope with GCE O and A levels. The majority of these students showed no knowledge of mental handicap, had obviously never thought about it, and held views and expectations obviously based on the most extreme and bizarre degrees of subnormality. They expected that their parents would react adversely to the foundation of a hostel in their area, and justified this attitude by the supposed danger the mentally handicapped present to children and old people. Confusion between the mentally handicapped and the mentally ill was also very common.

Ignorance and prejudice are not confined to the populace at large but may readily penetrate the kin group. One of the South London mothers, for example, expressed a great deal of bitterness at the way the whole of her immediate family had suffered. They felt that they had been cut off from their wider family and from friends and the community:

> Let's put it this way, there were relations we have not seen since we found out about Trevor ... [and] we have only been invited to tea with Trevor once to my brother-in-law. He thinks we should put Trevor away.

One justification for community care of mentally handicapped children, even if looking after them at home does lay a heavy burden on their mothers, is that they are thereby enabled to mix normally with other children and become assimilated into the normal life of the community. This was indeed a frequent outcome in our new city study, and where it occurs it forms an important and highly desirable part of the child's life. As with other children, not all make friends easily. In half of the families in our sample the children were described as 'not involved' with local children, or not interested in mixing with them, or in two cases as positively rejected by them, or else as having few opportunities to mix. (The 'mild' cases, surprisingly, seemed to be a trifle overrepresented in this group.) In the other cases, however, neighbours and neighbouring children did play a very important part in the handicapped child's life. Involvement tends to be most intense, as one might expect, in small village communities:

> He chucks his wheelchair around the street and everyone knows him, he goes in next door and has an hour in there and a cup of tea and biscuits, and then he goes off down the road, the old people love him ...
>
> The wheel came off his wheelchair the other day, and a little tot ... said 'Come quick, Edward's wheel has broken off his chair!' Well, I flew up ... and there were these five little tots, none of them were more than six (and he is a weight) and they had got it like this, and holding it so that he wouldn't go down. And their little faces! They really take care of him.

Urban life is also not incompatible with local involvement:

> At the moment she's in love with the boy next door. He's 16 and he's a nice lad, he takes an interest in her.

Even a blind and immobile child can benefit from local involvement:

> [Her sisters'] friends come in and out. I think most of their friends are better with her than the grown-ups. Irene's ... got a friend ... orange hair one side and bright green the other ... If you saw her in the street you'd think, 'What a terrible child!' She'll come in here and she'll pick her up and she laughs and giggles and she's absolutely marvellous. But I find that all the teenagers and even younger ... are very, very good. It's as they get to our age ...

It is of course true, however, that the converse of assimilation will also occur, and the often adverse reactions which families experience from relatives and from the general public are one key definer of the world in which the mentally handicapped child lives. Reactions range from neutral or even highly supportive (the latter particularly from the grandmothers of the children) to expressions of hostility, curiosity and distaste. One important point to note is that the parents of the mentally handicapped are of course themselves born members of the culture which despises their children, and they themselves carry these attitudes into their present situation. They may share them, or more likely fight them, or try to side-step them by aggressively declaring that their child is 'normal', but they cannot escape them; how they see their own situation is shaped, posit-ively or negatively, by cultural norms. Indeed, to bring the argument round full circle, the reactions which they perceive others as making may be supplied at least in part and on occasion by their own expectations. The point is well illustrated in an interview with one mother in the South London sample:

> When I talk to people and I say, 'Mark is mentally handicapped', and as soon as they know he is coming up to 16, you see, you know what I mean? I don't want to put it into words, but you see it before they even say it . . . It is an unspoken look. I suppose maybe I would be guilty in the same way, but there is that fear of danger to 'my daughter'.

However, even here the fact that the parents share, at some level, the same stigmatizing stereotype as they purport to recognize in others may be responsible at least in part for creating the problem – the parents may be oversensitive, or may even project into the situation their own unac-knowledged fears and feelings of distaste (see also Bayley 1973: 240).

Thus having a mentally handicapped child and caring for him or her at home presents the child's parents with two major tasks which are not faced in the same way by parents of 'normal' children. They have to come to terms with the fact of the child's handicap and its implications for the way in which the family is able to conduct its normal life in interaction with others. At the same time they have to deal with the way our society labels and stigmatizes mental handicap – including the way that the historically determined stereotype of mental handicap spills over as a courtesy stigma for the whole family – and this means renegotiating the nature of the family's identity and building a style of life compatible with the renegotiated identity. This task is made none the easier by the fact that the parents are themselves members of the culture which stigmatizes them and their children, may project their own feelings of spoilt identity onto the world at large and share to some extent the very attitudes which they are forced to combat.

The mother's life

The work of community care, despite genuine assistance received in some cases from the family, the community and the state, tends to fall over-whelmingly on the mother. Similarly, despite the effects of handicap on the whole nuclear family which have been documented above, it is the mother's life and life opportunities which are most disrupted by having a mentally handicapped child. The extent of the burden will of course vary from family to family; very different lives and experiences are in-cluded under the one arbitrary label of mental handicap. When the chil-dren are very young they may not present a burden of care any greater than the norm, unless there are coexistent physical problems: 'children are wonderful anyway', and Down's syndrome babies and some of the mildly retarded are particularly quiet, sweet and undemanding as infants. The 'parenting style' adopted may not be very different from that consid-ered appropriate for the other children in the family (which demonstrates how little the discoveries of educators and therapists percolate through to the family level – see Carr 1975: 827). The degree of extra work may not be apparent to the mother herself because it has become 'just part of the routine'. In her survey of Scottish families, Hunter (1980) asked the ques-tion, 'How does having a handicapped child affect your family?' and received from one mother the answer, 'It's not until somebody asks you about it that you realise what you have to do.' We had a similar experi-ence with our own research; an interim paper was discussed at a parents' meeting and the response to the section on the work of motherhood was that they had not realized until they saw it written out just how hard they did work. Nonetheless this labour and the need for it does exist, and the work falls predominantly on the child's mother.

Mothers of the mentally handicapped share with other mothers the substantial amount of work that bringing up any kind of child entails. The mentally handicapped child requires very much more labour over a lifetime, however. The work itself will generally be more intense. For example, all children are incontinent when they are young, but mentally handicapped children are incontinent for longer. Carr (1975) found that only 38 per cent of a sample of Down's syndrome children were 'clean and dry' by day by the age of 4, and only 18 per cent by night, compared with 88 per cent and 71 per cent respectively of an age-matched control sample. In a survey of Family Fund applicants (Bradshaw 1980) almost three-quarters of the 242 children over the age of 4 were still incontinent. Even 'mild' cases may not be trained until they are 4 or 5, and the most severely handicapped will be incontinent well into their teens, or forever. This means not only more years of cleaning up and extra washing, but much more to clean up – as the child grows older – and a heavier child to manoeuvre on and off the pot. Disturbance at night may also be a normal feature of life for these families for many years beyond the norm, and there may be no ready escape from it.

Worries about supervision form a second major load on mothers. Bradshaw (1980) found that nearly half of the parents who applied to the Family Fund for assistance considered that their children were at risk of harming themselves or others if left alone for any period of time, and only 27 per cent felt the child could be left to play alone. We found the same kind of emphasis among the mothers to whom we spoke. The con-sequences are time diverted from housework and from the other children, and a consequent extension of the 'houseworking day', sometimes late into the evening. If the mother needs to go out, even just for shopping, the more intensive child care which mentally handicapped children often require may make it difficult to find babysitters or child-minders or to persuade relatives to share the care. (Even if it were not in fact more difficult, the parents may think that it would be, and that in itself is just as restricting.) Even when the children are at school the mother may need to remain 'on call', and timings have to be very precise, with very little leeway in the schedule – 'I mean, you can't really leave a handicapped child really on its own.' The child must be met from the school bus – in some cases the driver will not leave the child if there is no one there waiting. School times come to dominate the lives of such mothers even more tyrannically than is normally the case:

> My life has been run by the school bus for 15 years now. You can't go out; you must be here. From the day these children are born your life is planned; you've got to put it around that child.

In the holidays the child cannot be left even for half a day unsupervised, so school holidays are very likely to mean dropping all other activities to go back 'on guard'. Moreover, as the quotation above indicates, the process is protracted far beyond the norm. Many mothers would not leave their 5-year-old child to come home from school to an empty house. Few, however, would still need to be there to receive a 15-year-old, with the prospect of still needing to be there when the 'child' is 25.

An important part of 'community care', as envisaged by its proponents, is the notion that 'the community' will support and sustain the family in its difficulties. Half of our new city sample did indeed receive considerable help from their neighbours, ranging from transport to hospital when needed or occasional babysitting to more crucial interventions. Two of the mothers were able to continue work when the children were still small because neighbours took care of them. Two more had neighbours on whom they could and did call in emergencies – for example, to meet the other children from school when the handicapped child had to be taken to hospital. One mother, indeed, was able to recruit a whole street of neighbours to apply an American training programme which calls for constant stimulation of the handicapped child. Eight families, however, did not know their neighbours or received little or no help from them. The kin-group, whether or not living in the immediate neighbourhood, was another important source of help or resources for some. Mothers, mothers-in-law, cousins and siblings provided money, transport for holidays, a warm place to take the baby from a cold flat, even the occasional 'weekend off'. Half of our sample, however, did not mention any degree of help from kin. In all, six of the 16 received help from neither the people living round them nor from their wider family, and in another five cases the help they received was comparatively trivial.

Even the help which is received from the nuclear family is not enough to change mothers' burdens appreciably. Eight mothers in our study mentioned minor help delivered by the siblings of the handicapped child – domestic work, or minor help with child care, or in one case babysitting. One mother, a widow, received very substantial help from her eldest son. Among the fathers, five are described as helping with child care – significant help in four cases. The contribution of six of them was not mentioned in either interview, which suggests they do as much or as little as most husbands. Five are described as doing little or nothing:

> Derek's not the sort of dad that does a lot, not knocking Derek, but I think he's an ideal man not to have kids.

> Harry has never been like a dad should be . . . He was very possessive, very possessive, but he never did anything to help me with him. I mean, he didn't walk till he was 4. And never did he ever think of carrying him upstairs . . . well, he never done anything for him. That was a woman's job.

Thus some help is received from the surrounding community or from the kin group or indeed from within the nuclear family, but in general it is not enough to normalize the lives of the mothers who are caring for mentally handicapped children. Help from the family or from outside may carry one through an emergency or make mother's life easier or more pleasant. Nonetheless it is mother who bears the responsibility of care; others only 'help'. (Three of our mothers, indeed, mentioned no such help at all in either interview, and in two others the nuclear family was the only resource.)

Returning to a full-time job within a year or so of the birth is 'of course' out of the question for mothers of mentally handicapped children, as it appears to be for mothers of many 'normal' children (see next section). In our sample of 16 mothers, for instance, none was currently in full-time paid employment, though all had worked before marriage. Seven had current employment of some sort – six in part-time or evening jobs, and one as a home-worker – and nine were not in employment at all. (Of this last group, however, two were already over 60.) This kind of pattern of substantially less involvement with paid employment than is the norm even for other married women is borne out by a number of other studies (see, for example, Bayley 1973; Glendinning 1983). The inability to take full-time paid employment matters a great deal, because women work not only for the money (important though that may be) but also for the social contacts that 'going to work' brings and the increased social status which being engaged in paid employment brings in a society which devalues the domestic role.

Many of the reasons given for going down to part-time employment or giving up an outside job altogether in our study were such as might be given by any mother, whether or not her child was labelled as handicapped: the burden of child care, the need to be at home when the children come home from school, the difficulty of school holidays, the need to take leave when the children are ill. Some explicitly denied that the child's handicap was a factor. All but four had worked at some time since the birth of their children, in an occupation which fitted school hours; school canteen assistant was popular, as were part-time jobs in shops or offices (9 till 3.30), and some had worked evenings as a cleaner or on an assembly line. One or two had done child minding or short-term fostering, or run playgroups, and several had run Tupperware parties and the like. One or two had managed a full-time job at some stage, but only because alternative child care was available. This kind of work pattern is fairly typical of any group of mothers. As we have seen, however, the mothers of the mentally handicapped have additional problems with which to contend.

People seem to be able to cope with almost anything, and most of our mothers coped with their load from day to day, trying to make a normal life for themselves and their families. One might want to distinguish, however, between families where 'normality' predominated and those where 'coping' is a more adequate descriptive term. In the latter class would fall those who would regard themselves as trying to treat the handicapped child as normal but who are resigned to the fact that they cannot entirely succeed in doing so and that the child makes a great deal of difference to their lives. They are 'resigned' to having a handicapped child rather than accepting of it, insofar as the two can be distinguished – they shade into each other. Often the problems lie with the nature of the handicap. Some children may be prone to violent outbursts, for example, out of frustration at their inability to communicate or, more worryingly, for no detectable reason. Sometimes the problem is to do with family lifestyle, as in the case of the busy mother who has three other children and manages to hold down an evening job as well when she is not child minding or undertaking short-term foster care; the (mildly) handicapped child is just a cross which the family is resigned to bearing – loved and cared for, but a nuisance nonetheless. Sometimes a life which might have been comparatively easy is made difficult by the compounding pressure of other circumstances, as with Mrs Jones, a lady living on one of the rougher council estates, who appears from her own account and that of her husband to be suffering systematic persecution from a neighbouring family. In this 'coping' class we should also place Mrs Inglish, who is coping with life in general only with a great deal of social service support. Herself educated in a Special School, and having spent a period in a psychiatric hospital, she has seldom held down a job for long; she is divorced, and the social services have assumed the parental responsibility for her children. Nonetheless, she is one who is managing to cope with the day-to-day care of the child.

One should remember that classifying a mentally handicapped child as 'the' problem of a family is a social construction which may not be shared by the family itself. For all the mothers we talked to the mentally handicapped child was indeed a problem, but for some there was another child about whom they worried more. Mrs Jones, for example, appeared more worried about her eldest child, who had a spell of truanting from school in response to the bullying from neighbouring children which followed on his evident grief at his grandmother's death. Another mother had a child suffering from cystic fibrosis who required daily medical or nursing attention. Another had a child who had been 'teacher's pet' at a small village school and was not reacting at all well to his transfer to a larger secondary school in the new city. Mrs Inglish was far more worried by her elder son Keith than by the mentally handicapped child; Keith was a boarder at a school for maladjusted children, and he tended to beat her up and smash the furniture when he came home on holiday.

In four of our families 'adaptation' rather than just 'coping' might be said to have taken place; the child appears to play the same role in the family as a 'normal' child would do, and family life seems to proceed 'as normal'. (The distinction between this group and those who just cope is not a hard and fast one, however, and may be an artefact of what happened to 'come out' at particular interviews.) One middle-class lady who lived in one of the neighbouring villages, for example, used to work in an office until her child was born, went back to similar work when the child was 3, and now (in her 40s) does some work as a cook in the local school. She spends a great deal of time with her child and has to some extent 'built her life around her', but one has the impression that this would have been her pattern of life if the child had not been handicapped; she seems happy and settled. Another continued with part-time office work all the time she lived near relatives who could babysit, helped her husband for two years when he was running his own business, and is currently looking round for a part-time job which would involve her with children. She seems very close to and involved with both her children equally and to enjoy the life she has with them. Another lady with three children (one mildly retarded, and one with cystic fibrosis) presented herself in interview very much as a classic 'working-class mum'. She switched from full- to part-time factory work when she married, went over to working in the evenings when her first child was born, and switched again to cooking in a canteen when the others were born in order to be more available when they came out of school. The mentally handicapped child appears to have presented few problems once he was out of nappies and to be treated very much like her eldest, normal child. The fourth lady found she had to give up work to look after her children – apart from the odd cleaning job and running the occasional Tupperware party – because her husband's long and irregular hours of work as a self-employed carpet fitter meant that he could not take regular responsibility for them. At the end of her interview, however, she surprised herself by saying:

> I think family life is important, and I mean, we are a normal family. My cousin said that once. I thought it was a queer thing to say. She said, 'I like it because you don't treat Edith anything but normal', and I said, 'Well, how the hell am I supposed to treat her?' But I thought about it afterwards and I suppose I could see what she meant, she wasn't being funny. We don't go out of our way because I've got a backward child, we don't not do anything, we do everything that, in fact, a normal family does.

These were all cases of a normal, unremarkable adaptation to family life. In six of our 16 interviews, however, it is possible to detect a more exaggerated and systematic 'style' of adaptation. One mother, for instance, describes herself as very much enjoying married life and seeing children as an important and integral part of it. After school she worked in a shop, then took evening classes and became a clerk, but she gave up work when she 'fell for' her first child – a pre-marital but planned pregnancy. She has done odd jobs since – cleaning in the evenings, and lunch-time jobs – but she feels she could not take a settled job because of the handicapped child. However, she says she would not take a full-time job even if he were not there, because her other (older) child needs her at home. Another lady, Mrs Allinson, has not held a job since her handicapped daughter was born, and she very much enjoys not doing so; despite the amount of effort she puts into her life, she regards herself as something of a 'lady of leisure'. A third lady aspired to the same style. Talking of her early aspirations, she lists the chief one as 'just wanting to get married and have a family', and she says she looked forward to not working as a relief. However, she has found caring for her two children very hard work; only now that they both go out to school is she beginning to enjoy the leisure to which she had looked forward. The fourth started her working life in a factory, but she did not enjoy it and was glad to quit after she was married, when she 'fell for' her first child. She is beginning to think of taking some kind of part-time job, but that would be some considerable time in the future, as her oldest is only 6.

These women might be seen, perhaps, as 'having marriage as a career' rather than just as being married. Another 'career' which one might detect in two of the interviews is that of child minding. One lady, for example, had a family of five children spread over nine years and was then told she was very unlikely to be able to have any more. Eight years later, when she had supposed she was menopausal, she conceived 'by accident' and bore a severely brain damaged child. (She promptly had her seventh child, to provide him with company.) He is now 16, with an assessed mental age of about 5 but a 'social age' (we met him) which presents as very similar to his chronological age. She is now 60, and he is very much the companion of her old age, while she is probably his closest friend and companion.

> He has been a marvellous child, he has given me lots and lots of pleasure . . . He'll stay. He won't be any different to what he is now . . . By the time I do go . . . we're all long livers in my family . . . he'll have had a good life, as good as anyone could give him.

The second lady in this category says of herself that

> I've looked after young children all my life. I was always baby minded, taking them out for walks. Very baby minded person, when I was very young . . . that was my one aim in life, to have loads and loads of children . . . I like children, you know, I like to be surrounded by children.

Of the 'respite' weekends that have been arranged for her, when Gerry goes into a hospital, she says

> It has taken me an awful long time to part with her even for odd weeks . . . I didn't trust them, anyway, with her, to think that they could just automatically cope with her. So it's continuously on the phone every day, phoning up. It took me about – 4 she was the first time I let her go in – until 11 before I really knew who I was talking to.

That the reluctance to let her go was not just related to the quality of her care is emphasized later in the interview:

> *Husband*: You see, the first idea of relief care, whether it sounds harsh or not, was to get Lorna used to not having her around . . .

> The idea in the beginning was to take her for longer and longer periods, so that she wouldn't be dependent on Gerry. You know, she wouldn't run her life.
>
> *Wife*: I think I should be lost without her; because my whole life does centre around her.

This case also provides a good illustration of how one's 'world picture' may change over time and how 'motivation' may sometimes be shaped teleologically to validate an outcome which is judged inevitable. At the time of our first interview she very definitely appeared to see herself as a child-centred person whose future employment would be in child care or in the care of the elderly – at least in part as a substitute for the daughter around whom her life had been centred until now. She confirmed in the second interview, a year later, that this had indeed been her picture of herself at the time and that she would indeed still feel lost and without purpose when Gerry has to go – that she might even break down at that point. However, since the first interview she had taken and passed a typing course and had every hope that she might obtain an office job at some time in the future if jobs of any kind were to be had. She now regards her earlier picture of her future as at least in part a rationalization of the inevitable.

In summary, the mother of the mentally handicapped child carries the same burden as any other mother – the burden of child care. This may be willingly accepted or even sought out and planned for, but it is nonetheless a life-consuming role which leaves little time or space for individuality. In that sense these mothers' lives are 'normal' for women, statistically and in terms of role-expectation, but as remote from the lives of men as are most married women's lives. Over and above the 'normal' constraints of other mothers, however, these women live a life more closely packed with problems, and the problems go on for a substantially longer period. This is the non-financial cost of community care.

Comparison with the 'normal'

Shortly after the second interviews with mothers of mentally handicapped children, one of us conducted a series of interviews with a sample of mothers whose children had *not* been labelled as mentally handicapped, roughly matched for size of family and area of residence (which correlates well, in the new city, both with social class and with availability of 'social resources'). The sample is of course too small and haphazard to be representative of mothers in general – and a similar charge might be levelled at the sample of mothers of the mentally handicapped – but the two samples match closely enough for some tentative comparisons to be drawn. One can after all say little about what is distinctive in the experience of mothering mentally handicapped children except by comparison with the general experience of mothering.

Compared with our 'mental handicap' sample, very few of these mothers commented on the amount of work which having children around the house entails. Ten had no particular comment to make at all, except (in four cases) to say that they did not enjoy housework. Five, on the other hand, expressed positive pleasure in domestic work. For example:

> I'm just that kind of person, I like to be tidy ... I like to do everything ... so that when I come home all I have to do really is tidy up in general down here, and give them a good cooked meal.
>
> (Mrs Blacker)

> People I know sit around and say 'I get bored', but I don't honestly get time. If I'm not gardening I'm decorating and if I'm not decorating I'm making – I do all my own dressmaking. If I'm not dressmaking I'm embroidering or knitting. Oh yes, I make the wine, I do the lot.
>
> (Mrs Greene)

> Washing their clothes, cooking for them, that's not hard work because it's a natural thing.
>
> (Mrs Royal)

Another lady described how she managed to render housework interesting by treating it as a nine-to-five job on the one hand and never letting it settle into an exact routine on the other. Only four people commented on the strains of the housewife's work, and their comments were to do mostly with how little sleep one seems to have during the first few years of a child's life.

One could well form the impression, in contradistinction to the mothers of mentally handicapped children, that these mothers did not regard the daily and yearly grind of motherhood as particularly hard work. This may to an extent be true; while mothering ordinary children is undoubtedly hard work, as anyone will testify who has children in the house, it is equally undoubtedly not as much work as mothering most mentally handicapped children. It differs in two other ways as well: (1) the children of these mothers were often of similar chronological ages to the children who appeared in the last section, but for this reason they were mostly more advanced in terms of development – the messier and heavier work lay in the past – and (2) the work entailed by a normal child has a foreseeable termination, which often means that it seems less onerous. It may be also that mothers underrate the work of being a housewife precisely because it is 'normal', taken for granted by everybody concerned, while the mothering of a mentally handicapped child leads one to think about the work involved. Two other factors should also be considered, however. First, our sample underrepresents women in full-time paid employment, which could well make a difference – though the two women in our sample who were in full-time employment were not among the ones who commented on the pains of housework. The second factor is that the interviewer was male; it is possible that different things might have been said to a female interviewer.

As regards help with the work, we formed the impression from the interviews that the mothers of the unlabelled children received much the same help and support from kin, but more from neighbours, than did the mothers of the mentally handicapped children – that they were more closely integrated into the local community. Of the 19 that we interviewed, 12 can be described as receiving (or having received in the past, when the children were younger) a fair amount of help from kin or neighbours or both, and another two as having received occasional or emergency help. The parents and/or parents-in-law of six of the families lived in the neighbourhood, and four of them had received a good deal of help with child rearing or child care. One has a sister who takes the children overnight, and another a mother who advises and provides practical help (and nieces who babysit whenever required). Mrs Scarlett stayed with her mother for a few days after her second child was born, to give her time to recuperate while not interfering with her husband's ability to work. Another of these ladies would say that her family were not on the whole a great source of help, but her mother has been over once or twice a week during the current pregnancy, to do housework and ironing and anything else that she judged too much of a strain for a pregnant woman. Two others did not see much of their parents now, but they were a great source of help before they moved from London to the new city. For example, when Mrs Forrest's first child was a baby her husband's parents lived just round the corner, and her own were only seven miles away, so babysitting was never a problem and they were able to go out – in the evening or during the day – whenever they wanted to do so. (With her later children she has been more restricted in that respect, but her parents come up for the weekend not infrequently, and Mrs Forrest and her husband generally take advantage of the situation.) Six informants out of the 19 rarely saw their parents or received little help from them, and seven had little or nothing to say about kin, but for six the 'extended family' was an important resource. This is much the same picture as emerged from the analyses in the last section – round about a third receiving significant help from the extended family.

A different picture emerges when we look at involvement with neighbours and the local community. Eight of the mothers of mentally handicapped children said they received little or no help from their neighbours, but only five of the mothers of unlabelled children were in this position. Seven of the 19 had a great deal of help from their neighbours – invaluable help in some cases, making the desired lifestyle possible rather than impracticable.

> The neighbours are super . . . I've always had a babysitter . . . If I want to go to bed at 10 in the morning and I've worked [on the night shift] the night before, my daughter gets her little shopping bag and goes off down [to a neighbour] . . . and goes with them to school . . . You just couldn't do these things without neighbours.
>
> (Mrs Whiting)

Four others mentioned occasional help, and two help in emergencies. Overall only five of the mothers of unlabelled children had little or no help from either kin or neighbours, and twelve had a great deal of help from one or the other or both. In comparison, eleven of the mothers of mentally handicapped children received either no help at all or only trivial assistance.

As regards help from within the nuclear family, six of our informants' husbands are described realistically (we checked by asking what they actually did about the house) as taking a share or doing a great deal. For example:

> Whoever comes in first starts the dinner. You do the cooking [to her husband] and some of the cleaning. I think you have to, because we both go out now, doing different things.
>
> (Mrs Olivier)

> My husband does housework, he's tidier than I am, actually. The other night I was out . . . I didn't get home till 10, and there he was ironing. He always bathes the kids . . . He can cook dinner. I went to France on a day trip . . . and he had the children all day, and his Dad, he was out of hospital for the weekend . . . he cooked them a dinner and took them to the park.
>
> (Mrs Blacker)

> I suppose it's because I hate [housework] that they all do their bit, even the 5 year old does a bit around the house . . . The oldest boy cooks the dinner if ever we're not there . . . [My husband] probably does more than I do, to be honest. I think he always has probably done more . . . because we've both always worked . . . If it came to say who is really boss in the kitchen, he would be . . . Two weeks out of three he does the shopping . . . He probably taught me most of what I know about cooking anyway . . . He'll do anything and everything around the house.
>
> (Mrs Whiting)

> I don't very often ask him to now, but when I had the children . . . he did ironing and different things . . . If I'm not well . . . he'll just come in and take over. When we were first married and both working, he'd come in and maybe wash up while I hoovered and things like that.
>
> (Mrs Forrest)

Another lady described how her husband will take over getting the supper and send her up to have a bath, when he gets in from work, if he thinks she looks under the weather, and how he has done her evening cleaning job once or twice when she has been ill. Seven others describe their husbands as doing a bit about the house – child care (3) or housework (1) or both (3) – but only in the sense of 'helping'. Six others described their husbands as offering little or no daily help. Adding these in, this still leaves three families where the wife receives virtually no help in keeping up the house and looking after the children, from nuclear family or kin or neighbours. The same number were without help in the families with mentally handicapped children.

Overall, then, the mothers of the unlabelled children and the mothers of the mentally handicapped children had much the same resources to draw on in their 'home work', with the exception that the mothers of unlabelled children seemed to receive more help from the surrounding community. One should not overrate the amount or quality of the help, however, in the majority of cases. While a few of our informants praised their husbands for the amount of work they did around the house and/or with the children, in only two cases were they prepared to say that the husband did as much (or more) as they did themselves, or that they could relinquish responsibility for the work. This is the general finding of research into husbands' involvement in the work of the home. Men may on occasion be substantially involved in child care – and perhaps increasingly so – but seldom in the remaining work of the house (though if mothers are asked not which tasks the husband undertakes but how often he undertakes them or how many hours he spends on them, it turns out that nearly 50 per cent of married men with children can best be described as only minimally involved in child care – see Boulton 1983). As regards housework, Edgell's 1980 study suggests that virtually no husbands take an equal share, and nearly half do virtually none. The families whom we have interviewed do not seem to be as extreme – there were a few cases of genuine help, within the limitation of work constraints – but we also formed the impression that most women none-theless receive precious little help in the day to day running of the house, and certainly that the running of the house remains the woman's respons-ibility in the vast majority of cases.

In this context, Backett (1982: 221) has pointed out in relation to her study of couples in an Edinburgh suburb that:

> In order for couples to sustain belief in [high] levels of father involve-ment they did not see it as necessary for him to participate fully or constantly. Rather it is a matter of each couple negotiating the kind of practical proof which they found to be subjectively satisfactory. This was done by the father's participating sufficiently regularly in those particular spheres which spouses had identified as being relev-ant to their own family situation.

She also points out that the situation for men is fundamentally different from the situation for women, where the man goes out to work and the wife stays at home. When the husband is at home, even if he were literally to take an equal share of available 'home work', it is a share; his wife is there to carry the other half. Thus a man may 'do' child care, or housework, and be fully committed to it. Never or seldom, however, is he faced with the daily problem that his wife faces when he is not at home – that both housework and child care have to be coped with at one and the same time.

In the sample of 16 mothers of mentally handicapped children, de-scribed in the last section, none was in full-time paid employment at the time of the interview. Six were in part-time or evening jobs, one was a home worker, and nine were not working at all. Of our sample of 19 mothers whose children were not labelled as mentally handicapped, two were in full-time employment (a proportion which undoubtedly under-rates the proportion in the population – those we approached who were in full-time employment tended to decline the interview), six were in a substantial part-time job, two did some part-time paid work and some voluntary work, one was substantially involved in voluntary work (as a Women's Institute county organizer), and three others did a small amount of part-time work or home work and helped out at their children's schools. Only five were in no form of employment, and one of those was in a late stage of pregnancy. The two groups differ substantially on this variable, therefore; the mothers of mentally handicapped children were markedly less able to take outside employment.

However, we should note that the presence of children in the home still made a substantial difference to the pattern of employment. Of those who worked full-time, one was on the night shift (as a nurse) so that there was always someone in the house to look after the children. Of the eight who were in part-time employment, six had jobs deliberately chosen to leave them free to be home when the children came home from school (morning work in a garage office, daytime shifts as a nurse, or the jobs in canteens or as school welfare officers which are so popular with mothers). There were no cases of men similarly curtailing their work patterns in the interests of the children. The responsibility for the children's welfare still falls disproportionately on the mothers.

Other factors which were evident in the 'mental handicap' interviews were far less salient in the other ones. Mothers of mentally handicapped children talked a great deal about the difficulties of being tied to the timetable of the child, which was a minority response among the other mothers interviewed; the unlabelled children remained children in that sense for a much shorter period before they could be trusted to look after themselves to some limited extent. The initial adaptation to the child was of course a major theme in the interviews with mothers of mentally handicapped children and not in the others, though there were a few comments about the difficulty of adapting to the lack of freedom (and of sleep!) which young children entail. Most noticeable was the relative absence in the interviews with mothers of unlabelled children of comments about the longer-term adaptations which the family had undergone and of the family's plans for the future. It seemed taken for granted in the majority of cases that having children was a temporary phase, though of long duration, yet on the other hand there was relatively little conscious planning for the future. One had the impression more of a state of faith that the future would take care of itself in a relatively unproblematic way, 'as it does for everybody else'.

The family's future

In the normal course of things children grow from babies to toddlers, go to school and become increasingly independent in their lives; they leave school, find a job (or, increasingly, fail to do so) and eventually cease to be the responsibility of their parents. As we have seen, mentally handicapped children generally go through the early stages of this life-course more slowly than others and thereby create substantial burdens which generally fall on their mothers. In their adolescence, however, they may constitute a substantial problem for both parents, because for some of them there is every likelihood that they will never leave home at all unless their parents make specific arrangements to send them away. As Dickerson and Brown (1978) have pointed out, the parents have one child who is not going to release them from responsibility. It gets to be a very big worry. Who is going to support this child? Who will pay the bills? Provide him a good home? Supervise his leisure time? . . . Keep him out of trouble? . . . The parents find that they need to make long-term arrangements for the disabled child in the event of their deaths.

In the shorter term, the children leave school at some time in their teens and may therefore no longer be off their parents' hands during the day.

One of the problems is that handicapped children grow less wonderful as they grow older. What was acceptable appearance and behaviour in someone who looks 5 or 10 years old may no longer be acceptable in someone who looks 20 or 30. Several of the mothers in the South London sample commented on this problem, and one had even had her daughter institutionalized to avoid the expected problems:

> This is one reason why something would have to be done. She went into the hospital . . . when she was 21. Caroline was 3 and Michael was 19, coming up to 20. I have seen so many families where the brothers have girlfriends and this causes unpleasantness, and . . . I said we have got to do something before Michael starts going serious with girlfriends, before Caroline goes to school and brings friends home. We don't want to make any unpleasantness.

At the same time, the mentally handicapped child may paradoxically become relatively younger – more of a burden to the family – in proportion as he or she becomes older physically. Even if no more of a burden, the 'child' remains the same burden for year after year in a 'frozen' family which has lost the space to change and in which the parents themselves are becoming older and less able to cope.

While the family's development is frozen, however, social provision is not; the provision for a family with a handicapped child tends if anything to decline as the child grows past school age. The real 'community care' for mentally handicapped children who grow into mentally handicapped adults is that they follow the 'normal' pattern and leave home – for a hostel and sheltered work, for a farm community or a group home, or for a hospital. For most families the time when children leave home is in any case a 'crisis point', but for the families of the mentally handicapped it is likely in addition to involve great feelings of guilt, because the child is generally not leaving home 'naturally' but being 'pushed out'. In the 16 families we interviewed in the new city, only one mother saw her retarded child as likely to leave home and live a normal life; this was a mildly handicapped child of 14 who was already showing every sign of being able to cope adequately and whose retarded uncles were coping in the outside world. Six others thought their child would always stay at home with them, but half of these were also considering the possibility of placement in a hostel or a sheltered community when they became unable to cope. Two (whose children were aged respectively 8 and 5) had not considered the topic. The other seven were already beginning negotiations for a hostel place or a place in a residential school or community. Thus well over half of our sample had to deal in their minds with the possibility or the likelihood of handing care over to others, and of these seven were expecting or fearing that the care would have to be in some sort of institution. The very childishness which makes the child a burden at home and necessitates the arrangements for continuity of care, para-doxically, increases the stress and the guilt of relocation:

> When you think what her mental age is, say 4 or 5, by the time she's 19 it won't be much more than that. You wouldn't stick a 5-year-old in a hostel, would you?

The choice of a proper institution or facility and the battle to be accepted there – as funds, and therefore places, are limited – can be a problem before which all earlier problems seem trivial and manageable.

Conclusions

To recapitulate, then, we have looked in this chapter at the real costs of bearing and bringing up a mentally handicapped child in the community. Some of it – the day to day grind of 'child work' – falls largely on the child's mother, though her involvement in it has consequences for the rest of the family. The rearing of a mentally handicapped baby does not differ in kind from the rearing of any other baby – itself a substantial social burden – but it differs in its density and its duration. The care of a retarded child may require constant vigilance, and the lateness of nor-mal stages of development doubles or trebles the burden of an ordinary problem such as incontinence. The burden goes on, moreover, potentially forever, unless the decision is made to send the child away – to the point where aging parents can no longer cope or provision must be made for what happens after their death or in the case of their eventual incapacity. (The potential exceptions – at least three out of our sample of 16 – are those whose children are not expected to live beyond their 20s; some of the mental handicaps have coexistent physical problems of great sever-ity.) Specific to mental handicap, however, is the other major range of problems which families encounter: the reactions which the notion of mental handicap engenders in our culture, among strangers and also within the family and kin group. Not least of this range of problems is that the parents of the retarded are themselves a part of the culture which stereo-types retardation and have to cope with their own reactions and their expectations of how others will react as well as with the real situation.

References

Abbott, P. A. (1982) 'Towards a social theory of mental handicap'. PhD thesis, London: Thames Polytechnic.

Backett, K. C. (1982) *Mothers and Fathers: A Study of the Development and Negotiation of Parental Behaviour*. London: Macmillan.

Bayley, M. (1973) *Mental Handicap and Community Care*. London: Routledge & Kegan Paul.

Birenbaum, A. (1970) On managing a courtesy stigma. *Journal of Health*, 196–206.

Boulton, M. G. (1983) *On Being a Mother: A Study of Women with Pre-School Children*. London: Tavistock.

Bradshaw, J. (1980) *The Family Fund: An Initiative in Social Policy*. London: Routledge & Kegan Paul.

Carr, J. (1975) *Young Children with Down's Syndrome: Their Development, Upbringing and Effects on their Families*. London: Butterworth.

Cummings, S. T. (1976) The impact of the child's deficiency on the father: A study of fathers of mentally retarded and chronically ill children. *American Journal of Orthopsychiatry*, 46: 246–55.

Dickerson, M. and Brown, S. (1978) A search for a family, in S. Brown and M. Moersch (eds) *Parents on the Team*. Michigan: University of Michigan Press.

Edgell, S. (1980) *Middle-Class Couples: A Study of Segregation, Domination and Inequality in Marriage*. London: Allen & Unwin.

Gallagher, J. J., Beckman, P. and Cross, A. H. (1983) Families of handicapped children: Sources of stress and its amelioration. *Exceptional Children*, 50: 10–19.

Glendinning, C. (1983) *Unshared Care: Parents and their Disabled Children*. London: Routledge & Kegan Paul.

Goffman, E. (1963) *Stigma: The Management of Spoilt Identities*. Harmondsworth: Penguin.

Greengross, W. (1976) *Entitled to Love?* London: Marriage Guidance Council.

Hunter, A. B. J. (1980) *The Family and Their Mentally Handicapped Child*. Barnardo Social Work papers no. 12.

Shearer, A. (1972) *A Report on Public and Professional Attitudes Towards the Sexual and Emotional Attitudes of Handicapped People*. London: Spastics Society/National Association for Mental Handicap.

Tredgold, A. F. and Soddy, K. (eds) (1970) *Tredgold's Mental Retardation*, 11th edn. Eastbourne: Baillière, Tindall & Cox.

Walker, N. and McCabe, S. (1973) *Crime and Insanity in England*, vol. II. Edinburgh: University of Edinburgh Press.

FIVE

PLANNING RESEARCH: A CASE OF HEART DISEASE

Pamela Abbott

This chapter is concerned to explain how I and a colleague (Geoff Payne) made the decisions which we did make about the design and sample size for a survey that we are carrying out in collaboration with a District General Hospital in the South-west of England. Issues of research design and sampling are crucial to the credibility of the research findings. Mistakes and misjudgements made at this stage of the research programme are difficult if not impossible to rectify at a later stage. Textbooks on research methods tend to lay down definitive statements about research designs and sample sizes, while our own theoretical perspectives may lead us to prefer one style of research to another. However, as I shall show here, both theoretical preferences and textbook ideals have to be compromised when we are confronted with the 'real world' and are actually carrying out research in it. It is also essential to recognize that when research is commissioned the researcher is being employed as an expert in research. Those commissioning the research may have a political agenda, which may or may not be shared by the researcher. Provided the researcher does not have ethical objections to the purpose of the research, however, politics have to be kept outside the planning and conduct of the research. Just as we may believe such and such a hypothesis to be true but be required as researchers to design a study which allows the possibility that the hypothesis can be disproved, so we may hold a political position and have hopes for the outcome of a piece of research but are required to design it to allow the possibility that the opposite position could be upheld by it.

The request for us to undertake research was made by the consultant cardiac surgeon at a District General Hospital. He approached the Faculty of Human Sciences at Polytechnic South West, to explore the possibility of collaborative research. The design of the research, sampling and sample size were discussed fully with him at all stages of the planning process.

The specific problem which he wanted researched was the experiences of patients who had to travel to East London for open-heart surgery. The District General Hospital has no facilities for such surgery, and all patients, private and national health, have to travel to London. The journey time by public transport to the hospital in London is at least five hours for these patients, and considerably longer for those who live in the rural areas surrounding the urban area where the District General Hospital is located. The initial problem with which we were asked to assist was the investigation of how patients and their partners actually experienced the travel to and the stay in London. It was hoped that this would provide a basis for developing better ways of preparing patients and partners, and specifically that it would enable a booklet to be written that could be given to all patients referred to London. However, it quickly became evident that the consultant had a hidden agenda; he was obviously interested in obtaining evidence to use in a campaign to procure open-heart surgery provision at the District General Hospital, and he hoped the research would begin to provide a basis for evaluating patients' experiences of 'internal markets' within the NHS. For this reason we tried to design the research so that our politics did not influence the research process or dictate the outcomes.

The design of the research and the decisions on sampling size emerged over a period of time, as we became aware of the complex nature of the issues with which we were dealing. Initially I felt that this was a research area that necessitated a qualitative approach. My preference at this stage was for in-depth interviews with patients and their partners to explore in detail their experiences and to find out what additional help they would find beneficial. This would have enabled us to explore in depth how people actually experienced travelling to London. It would have given us a vivid picture of what happened, what they experienced and how they felt about it. An informal, naturalistic interview procedure would have encouraged them to provide frank and detailed information. However, the costs of such methods, in time and the small number of people that could be interviewed, made them impractical. We could have handled only a small sample of couples, and this may well have provided atypical accounts; we needed 'across-the-board' information to provide a basis for helping future patients and their partners. We therefore decided that we would design a questionnaire, with analysis being undertaken using SPSSx on computer. We tried to keep the questions as naturalistic as possible, however; that is, the questions dictate the subject matter of the response but do not delimit the range of responses. Given the wide geographical area from which patients travel to the District General Hospital, we thought at this time that we would use a postal questionnaire.

In order to design the questionnaire we decided that we needed to know more about the actual experience of patients and their partners. The consultant cardiac surgeon arranged for four former patients (two male and two female) who had travelled to London for surgery, and their partners, to come to the District General Hospital. Geoff Payne and I carried out an open-ended group interview, which was taped and transcribed. This was used to provide basic information for the design of the questionnaire. Drafts of the two questionnaires, one for patients and one for their partners, were sent out to these six people, and they were asked to complete them, to suggest any questions that they thought we should have asked and to give their comments. Copies of the questions we asked were also sent to the consultant and the ward sister on the cardiac unit for their comments. On the basis of their comments the questionnaires were amended. It also became evident that it would not be possible to use them as postal questionnaires, given the difficulties these patients reported in completing the questionnaires at home themselves, but that an interviewer would be needed. It was agreed that interviews could take place at the hospital when the patients were asked to come in for a routine examination.

The analysis of the transcribed material and consideration of what we wanted to find out – which was now a broader range of questions than just what was needed to compile an information booklet – also led us to realize that it was not sufficient to interview patients and their partners who had already been to the London hospital. First, it became evident that we needed to follow a sample of patients and their partners through the process – that is, to interview them before they went to London and after they or their partner had undergone surgery in London. This would enable us to gain a much better understanding not only of how people felt about the process and their actual experiences but also of the types of information and support that could be given. It was also evident from the transcribed group interview that we needed to separate out the specific problems and difficulties associated with travelling to London from their experience of undergoing a major operation which was perceived to be life-threatening, or of being the partner of such a person. We realized that we needed a comparison or control group. Ideally this group should be identical to our sample except that they or their partners did not have to travel a long distance to have surgery. The obvious choice initially would seem to be the local patients at the London hospital. However, on reflection we realized that not only would it be practically difficult for us in terms of carrying out the interviews, but the characteristics of the London population were very different from those of our South-west sample of England. This precluded that possibility of a time-constrained sample of all patients (which is what we were using as the South-west sample). It might have been possible to use a matched-pair design – selecting a patient in London who had the same characteristics as each patient from the South-west. However, this would have extended the length of the study by an unknown amount, and the London sample would of course have been untypical of London patients. A further complication was that we did not have the same facilities in London as we had negotiated in the District General Hospital to interview patients. We decided that we would have to use, as a comparison, patients who were treated at the local hospital who were undergoing a procedure of a similar nature and were likely to have comparable characteristics. The consultant cardiologist suggested that patients undergoing major aortic repair would be suitable in terms of the criteria we specified.

This meant we now had a research design that involved us in interviewing six groups of people:

1 Patients who had undergone heart surgery in London.
2 The partners of these patients.
  These were retained in the design, although formally redundant because the information is duplicated by Groups 3 and 4, because we needed data to get the information booklet out as quickly as possible, given that a before-and-after design takes considerably longer than retrospective research. In this case patients may have to wait some time

between referral to the hospital in London and the actual date of the operation. We would then have to allow them to return from London and recover (at least six weeks) before they were interviewed.

3 Patients who were referred for heart surgery to London (to be interviewed when first told of the referral, and after the operation).

4 The partners of such patients (also to be interviewed twice, at the same points).

5 Patients undergoing aortic repair at the District General Hospital (again interviewed before and after).

6 The partners of such patients.

The questionnaires for the six groups were designed on the basis of responses to the first two that had been developed and piloted. The coding frame for the analysis of the data when the interviewing was completed was developed at this stage as well. When the questionnaires for Groups 1–4 were prepared, we trained the interviewer. She then carried out a small number of interviews at the hospital, and on the basis of feedback from her, some minor modifications were made to the questionnaires. The six final versions were prepared and printed, using a different colour of paper for each questionnaire.

The other key issue was sample size. We wanted a large enough sample to be able to analyse the data using two and three-way tables – to be able to display the interaction of one variable with another taking account of a third (i.e. differences between partners and patients in terms of worries about the operation, controlling for social class or for age of patient), and to use a test of significance such as Chi-squared to check that the results were not likely to be random sampling variations. We also wanted, for the retrospective groups (Groups 1 and 2), to collect the information reasonably soon after the operation, because of the risk of memory loss or distortion. Given the reasons for the research we did not want it to extend over more than two years, including data collection, analysis and report writing. We also wanted the sample to be representative of people undergoing open-heart surgery in the area (a quite diverse group, as it turned out). About 200 NHS patients are referred from the area each year to the hospital in East London for open-heart surgery. (We excluded private patients because of the small numbers and because they are referred to a different London hospital.) We decided that this gave us an adequate sample size and fitted in with our timing. We would interview all patients who had undergone open-heart surgery in the previous 12 months and all those referred to London in the coming 12 months. A similar-sized sample of aortic repair patients would be interviewed at the same time.

So we had designed our research and decided on our sample size. Two additional elements were added at this stage. We decided that a simple stress questionnaire would be administered by a nurse as part of the routine procedures on admission to hospital for surgery – both for those in London who were going to have open-heart surgery and those in the District General Hospital who were having surgery to repair the aortic artery. This would enable us to determine if those patients travelling to London for major surgery showed more evidence of stress than those having surgery at the local hospital. We also decided that a researcher would travel to London on public transport with a small subset of the open-heart patients, to observe and to talk to them and the people travelling with them. This would give some qualitative data on how patients and their partners actually experienced the journey and being admitted to the hospital or finding accommodation convenient to it.

The research was designed so that we could provide information, when the data were collected, on the experience of travelling to London for surgery, the problems that people experienced and how they felt about it all. It was also designed so that we could determine what factors were attributable to travelling and what to the fact that the patient was about to have major surgery. It was aimed both at providing this information and to act as a basis for helping patients and partners to be better prepared and supported by the hospital staff in the South when they had to travel to London for surgery. At the point at which this chapter was written, field work had only just begun. However, the specific outcomes we expect are:

1 A practical booklet for patients and their partners, explaining to them what will happen and giving useful information.
2 Providing advice to nurses and doctors on how they can better prepare patients travelling to London for heart surgery (and possibly more generally to nurses and doctors caring for any patients who have to travel some distance for treatment).
3 Contributing to the debate on internal markets in the NHS.

SIX

HOME HELPS AND DISTRICT NURSES: COMMUNITY CARE IN THE FAR SOUTH-WEST*

Pamela Abbott

Introduction and background to the research

Research into community care has tended to focus on the role of informal carers – especially women – and the burdens that community care policies place on them. Less attention has been paid to the work undertaken by paid carers, especially those who provide day to day social and domestic care. This chapter details the findings of research undertaken into the 'skills mix' required in such work and focuses on the roles of the main formal carers, home helps and district nurses. Home helps and district nurses are the services most frequently provided to enable frail elderly and chronically sick or disabled people to remain in the community, but it is home helps that perform the basic social and domestic care tasks which are actually what enable such people to continue to live in the community, especially when they do not have an informal carer. District nursing teams provide for more specialized nursing needs, although both district nurses and home helps provide personal care. It is in delivering personal care that an overlap occurs between services provided by Social Services and Health Care Trusts, with the potential for boundary disputes between home helps and district nurses (Abbott 1994). District nurses tend to see home helps as unqualified and lacking skills, encouraging dependency and being unaware of when elderly people's frailty necessitates nursing supervision of personal care. Home helps, in contrast, see district nurses as distancing themselves from clients and seeing home helps as 'domestics' rather than treating them as colleagues providing shared care for clients. There are also questions of acceptability: are clients happy with having personal care tasks performed by home helps, for example?

Statutory services are provided for only a very small percentage of those aged 65 or older (see Table 6.1). About 7 per cent of those aged 65 or older have a home help (SSI 1987), rising to 30 per cent of those aged 85 or older (OPCS 1986). Twenty per cent of people aged 65 or older are visited by a district nurse during the course of the year – about 6 per cent at least once a month. Of those aged 75 or older about 6 per cent attend a day centre, and 1 per cent have a day hospital place. Three per cent of people aged 65 or older have meals on wheels, but 5 per cent of those aged 75

Table 6.1 Use of home care services in Great Britain by people aged 65+, during previous month (1985)

	Age group	
	65–74 (%)	75+ (%)
Home help	4.2	13.5
Home nurse	3.5	8.4
Day centre lunch club	6.9	7.1
Meals on wheels	0.8	5.1

Source: adapted from OPCS (1986)

or over and 11 per cent of those aged 85 or over do. (OPCS 1986). However, for those who receive these services they are essential in enabling them to remain in the community in their own homes.

Domiciliary services in Cornwall

The research on which this chapter is based was undertaken in Cornwall in 1992. Cornwall is a rural shire county in the far South-west of England; when allowance is made for population spread it has the lowest population density of any English county. It has a reputation as a retirement area – that is, people migrate to the area on retirement. It is therefore likely both that it will have a higher percentage of older people than many other parts of Great Britain and that more of them will be living at a distance from relatives. The 1990 FHSA Register gave a total population for Cornwall of 467,886. Of these, 49,525 were aged 65–74, 32,352 were aged 75–84 and 9,555 were 85 or older. Nineteen per cent of the population of Cornwall were aged 65 or older, and 2 per cent were aged 85 or older.

If service provision in Cornwall were the same as the national average, then 6,400 people aged 65 or older would have a home help, 18,286 would be visited by a district nurse during the course of a year, and 2,743 would receive meals on wheels. In fact the Home Help Service in Cornwall is providing for about 4,500 people per year, and meals on wheels are distributed to about 1,500 people a year. The Council provides or pays for 680 day care places per week for the elderly. At the time of the research, services for the elderly consumed just over a seventh of Cornwall Social Services' annual budget (Cornwall Social Services, undated). The Social Services also made provision for 20,300 physically handicapped people, of whom 75 per cent were aged 65 or older. The Cornwall and Isles of Scilly Health Authority reported in 1989 that 60 per cent of its budget was spent on the 65 and over age group, who occupied 25 per cent of hospital beds and were twice as likely to visit their GPs as people in younger age groups.

The low population density of Cornwall, combined with the high proportion of elderly people, results in special problems of service delivery. The problems are especially acute in rural areas:

1 Isolation, especially of immigrants who may not have local friends or relatives.
2 The cost of service delivery, in terms of car mileage and the travel time of staff.
3 The high cost and low availability of transport for frail elderly people, which is particularly a problem in providing day centre care (Lennon 1991).

Health and social services, both statutory and voluntary, tend to be concentrated in towns. Those in rural areas tend to be deprived of transport, and this is a two-way problem, in terms of both service delivery and access to services.

In Cornwall, as elsewhere in Britain, the majority of care is provided by informal carers – relatives and friends. In addition, the voluntary sector – especially WRVS (the Women's Royal Voluntary Service) and Help the Aged – and the private (commercial) sector are important. Statutory services are provided by the FHSA (GPs, dentists and pharmacies), the Health Authority, Cornwall Community Health Care Trust and Cornwall Social Services Department. The services provided by the plethora of carers are both complementary and overlapping. At the time of the research it was felt that lack of co-ordination among service providers could result in clients not receiving services that could have been of benefit to them or receiving the same service from more than one agency.

Service providers in three GP practices

Three GP practices were selected to provide a focus for the research. Practice 1, 'Markettown', is located in a small market town in the east of Cornwall. It serves a large rural hinterland, and service provision is concentrated in the town. Practice 2, 'Porttown', is in a small coastal port and Practice 3, 'Village' is in a village, both in the west of Cornwall. Users in Porttown and Village received district nursing services from the same team, which was based in a small town (hereafter 'Smalltown'). Meals on wheels were delivered to both areas from Smalltown, and day-care provision was also located there. The home help service for Porttown was also based in Smalltown, but Village's provision was based in the village itself. Home help organizers for both were based some 20 miles away. While the distance from Porttown and Village to Smalltown is not large (5–10 miles), the population in both areas is scattered and public transport facilities are poor.

The range and type of community care services available to users in all three GP practices are broadly similar and comprise informal, voluntary and private (commercial) as well as statutory services. Four main groups are involved in providing community care: 'informal' carers, voluntary workers, the commercial sector and the statutory agencies. The main statutory providers of domiciliary care, numerically, are home helps and members of the District Nursing Team.

In Cornwall, as in many other parts of England, the work undertaken by the home help service has changed in recent years. Home helps mainly provide a service for frail elderly people considered to be at risk of admission to residential care. Only those who need help with social care (shopping, meal preparation and cooking, collecting pensions, etc.) and/or personal care receive a home help. Home helps continue to do domestic work, but only as part of a package of care.

All clients who were identified as users by the district nursing team leader and/or the senior home help in the three GP practices in October 1991 were interviewed in their own homes. In addition, interviews were carried out with seven people who were patients of one of the three practices and attended the day hospital. If an informal carer was living at the same address he or she was also interviewed. District nurses and home helps also completed a questionnaire specifying what tasks they performed for each client and their perceptions of their role. I also accompanied home helps and members of the district nursing team when they visited clients. This gave me an opportunity not only to talk to them informally but also to observe the work they undertook and the ways in which they interacted with clients. It also gave me the chance to chat informally with clients. Subsequently, district nurse team leaders and home help organizers completed a questionnaire designed to elicit information on who was responsible for care tasks for clients in different circumstances. This element of the research used vignettes (see Abbott and Sapsford 1983, reproduced as Chapter 7 of this volume).

Clients in the three areas

In total 100 clients were interviewed – 32 men and 68 women. Eight per cent were aged 16–64 and chronically sick or disabled, 21 per cent were between 65 and 74, and 71 per cent aged 75 or over. The analysis below is based on their responses, but not all clients answered every question. Fifty-three were visited by the district nurses and 54 by the home helps; 42 had only a home help, 40 only a district nurse and 11 had both services. Forty-eight clients had someone living with them (16 in Markettown and 32 in Porttown and Village). Forty-six said they had a main carer, while 61 said they had an informal carer who helped them with daily tasks. Sixteen of the main carers were male and 30 female. Thirteen of those who said they had a main carer also had a home help: eight where the main carer was male and five where the carer was female. The majority of the carers were themselves over 75 years, and only a quarter were under the age of 60. A spouse was the most likely person to be a main carer; 63 per cent of those who had a main carer were cared for by their spouses. Only a small minority had a carer who was not a close relative (see Table 6.2). A majority of

Table 6.2 Relationship of informal main carer

Spouse	29	(63%)
Daughter/in-law	8	(17.5%)
Son/in-law	3	(6.5%)
Other	6	(13%)

Table 6.3 Services visiting in the last six months

	Persons living on their own			Persons living with others		
	Markettown	Porttown	Village	Markettown	Porttown	Village
Consultant	–	–	1	–	–	2
GP	20	6	7	12	13	8
Practice nurse[1]	–	–	–	–	5	–
Health visitor	–	–	–	1	1	–
District nurse	12	7	6	11	18	7
Community psychiatric nurse	1	1	–	–	–	–
Macmillan nurse	–	1	–	–	1	–
Home help	21	12	6	10	3	2
Paid helper	8	1	2	5	5	6
Social worker	3	1	1	4	3	–
Occupational therapist	2	–	1	3	5	3
Unpaid helper	6	3	3	2	1	–
Minister of religion	8	3	1	3	5	3
Other voluntary worker	2	–	–	2	2	2

Note: [1] The practice nurse in Porttown began to visit people over the age of 75 for health checks at the same time as we started interviewing.

the sample lived in owner-occupied housing. Eighteen per cent lived in sheltered housing – 11 per cent provided by the local authority, and 3 per cent privately – and eight per cent lived with relatives or friends.

We asked the users which of a range of informal, statutory and voluntary services had visited them in the last six months. The most frequently mentioned were GPs (66), district nurses (61) and home helps (54), and the least often seen were consultants, community psychiatric nurses and health visitors (see Table 6.3).

We asked those who did have an informal carer what tasks the carers performed for them. The main ones were domestic and social rather than personal and nursing care. Shopping was the task most frequently mentioned, and cleaning teeth and help in feeding were the least frequent (tasks required only by the most frail). Allowing for the difference in numbers, the tasks performed by male carers did not seem to differ from those performed by female carers to any great extent.

Fifty-two of the people interviewed said they had a paid private helper. Twenty-seven of these lived in Markettown and 25 in Porttown or Village. Of those living in Markettown, 15 had a home help, 10 were visited by the district nurse, and two received both services. In Porttown and Village eight had a home help, 11 received district nurse services and five were visited by both.

Fifty-four of the people interviewed said they saw a chiropodist regularly. Of these, 28 saw the local authority chiropodist and 26 had a private one. Four of those who saw a chiropodist went to a day centre, 26 had a home help, 19 received district nursing services, and five were visited by both district nurse and home help. Of those who did not visit a chiropodist, five had their feet looked after by a spouse.

People who lived alone were more likely to receive home help services

Table 6.4 Whether lived alone and visits by district nurses, home helps and informal carers

	District nurse visited		Home help visited		Informal carer visited	
	Yes	No	Yes	No	Yes	No
Whether lives alone						
Yes (%)	31	69	76	24	42	58
No (%)	69	31	30	70	7	93
Significance	$p<.01$		$p<.001$		$p<.001$	

(Chi-squared with one degree of freedom)

Table 6.5 Personal care tasks and who performs them, among clients visited by both district nurses and home helps

Task	District nurse only	District nurse and home help
Bathing	11	6
Dressing/undressing	3	1
Getting up etc.	2	–
Washing hair	5	–
Washing feet	8	3

and to be visited by informal carers than those who lived with someone else (Table 6.4). Those who had someone living with them were more likely to be visited by a district nurse.

Home helps and clients were asked what services the home help provided for them, from a list based on the job description in the home help book with some additional tasks home helps are said to perform for clients. There were some discrepancies between what home helps said they did and the services that were perceived by clients as being provided. The most frequently mentioned task was general housework, followed by social care tasks. Tasks less frequently mentioned were personal care tasks and taking clients to various kinds of places.

There were also discrepancies between the tasks the district nurses saw themselves as performing and those the patients thought they received. (The list of tasks was drawn up from the job description for all grades on district nursing teams.) The tasks most frequently mentioned by nurses were advising patients about accidents in the home (76 per cent), providing advice about aids (37 per cent) and washing feet (58 per cent). No patient said that he or she had been given advice about using aids, only six (15 per cent) of those visited by a district nurse said they had been given advice about accidents, and 11 (27 per cent) said the district nurse washed their feet. Personal as opposed to nursing care tasks were more likely to be performed for patients by district nurses in Porttown and Village than in Markettown. A majority of patients receiving personal care from nurses were *not* also visited by home helps.

A majority of users received only one service, but a small number were provided with more than one. In some cases this was because a very specialized service was being received; examples here would be patients cared for by district nurses who were also visited by Macmillan nurses or Geriatric Liaison nurses. In other cases the services were clearly complementary – for example, meals on wheels provided on days when clients did not have home care.

Even if we examine the cases where clients were visited by both district nurses and home helps, there seems to be a clear division of tasks. In the majority of cases the interview and observation data suggest that the district nurses were carrying out specialized nursing tasks and the home helps personal care tasks. Observation of the district nurses in Porttown and Village suggests that they carry out personal care tasks for shared-care clients on days or at times when the home help was not visiting. District nurses did a high proportion of baths in Porttown and Village, including all those where lifting was required. In Markettown, where there were no auxiliary nurses in the district nursing team at the time of the research, most personal care, including baths, was done by home helps. However, the district nurses were concerned about the ability of the home helps to do personal care and the home helps felt that they were not recognized as part of the care team by the district nurses.

Informal carers performed a wide range of tasks, except the most specialized. Only 13 people who said they had a main carer also had a home help. (Indeed, one case was reported to me of an elderly man having his home help service withdrawn when his 18-year-old grandson moved in with him.) Observation and interviews with the home help organizers and senior home helps indicated that in general these carers were themselves frail and elderly. District nurses provided specialized nursing care where there is a carer present, as well as personal care in some cases.

In theory, clients could pay privately for any of the tasks performed by the statutory services. The main private service used by those interviewed was chiropody, often in order to get a home visit to have toenails cut. Private helpers were generally employed to carry out tasks such as gardening and household repairs which are not provided by the statutory services. A small number of users had paid helpers. For example, one district nurse patient paid for help with personal care, and two home help clients paid a helper to do shopping. Five home help clients paid to have laundry done, and three paid someone to do general housework. Thirteen home help clients paid for help with meal preparation and cooking, and one paid someone to bring in the food. In a small number of other cases where a user was paying someone to do domestic or social care tasks they received district nurse services but no home help.

District nursing services

All members of district nursing teams who visited patients attached to the three target GP practices were accompanied on some of their visits and sent a questionnaire about the work that they do and their attitudes to it. In total 16 questionnaires were sent out and 11 replies were received. All were asked which of a list of nursing and personal care tasks they performed for at least one patient; the list included a wide range of tasks spanning personal and medical/nursing care, including health education. All the tasks we listed were performed by at least one member of the team for at least one patient by nurses serving Porttown and Village, with the exception of taking blood.

Personal care tasks (making and changing beds, lifting patients in and out of bed and to the toilet, hair care, nail care, shaving, assistance with mobility) were performed by all members of the team; the qualified nurses undertook specialized nursing tasks in addition. In Markettown a number of personal care tasks were *not* performed for any patient – strip washes, bagging incontinence pads for collection, assisting patients with mobility outside the home, lifting patients in and out of the bath, and making and changing beds. Other personal care tasks – helping patients to undress and/or wash, bathing, applying incontinence pads, emptying commodes, hair care and the administration of medicine (tablets) – were done only by the state registered nurse who worked evenings. This appeared to be related to the fact that no auxiliaries were employed (see Chapter 7 of this volume).

The district nurses were asked if they ever performed tasks for patients that were not part of the nursing care plan. All except one said that they did. The tasks mentioned generally related to nursing care and included collecting dressings, equipment and prescriptions, assessment visits and giving general advice and support, making cups of tea or coffee and occasionally making breakfast if the patient was unwell. Other tasks mentioned by one or more district nurses included taking in the milk and the post, advice on filling in forms, changing light bulbs, washing underwear, occasionally lighting a fire, and putting dirty linen in to soak. Overall, however, few tasks were performed for patients on a regular basis that were not part of the nursing care plan.

All members of the district nursing team were visiting some patients who were also clients of the home help service and regarded at least some of these as having shared care. All of the nurses bar three regarded themselves as having regular contact with the home helps, though one qualified this by saying that it was only on a casual basis. Eight of the respondents were visiting patients for whom they and the home helps performed the same tasks. The tasks mentioned were all personal care tasks, washing and dressing being the most frequently mentioned. In six of the eight cases the patients concerned also needed specialized nursing care. All of the members of the district nursing teams except three said that they visited patients who required only help with personal care – assistance with bathing/shaving, getting up and dressed, and getting undressed and going to bed.

The home help service

A questionnaire was sent out to all the home helps and senior home helps with clients who were on the lists of the three GP practices. In addition, questionnaires were sent to home helps in Smalltown. Thirty-seven questionnaires were sent out and 31 returned (Table 6.6). All except two of the

Table 6.6 Response rate to the home help questionnaire

Location	Questionnaires sent out	Questionnaires returned			Per cent returned
		Home helps	Senior home helps	Total	
Markettown	14	10	–	10	71
Porttown	9	6	1	7	78
Village	7	6	1	7	100
Smalltown	7	6	1	7	100

Table 6.7 Average hours per week worked by home helps and senior home helps in four locations

Hours	Markettown	Porttown	Village	Smalltown	Total
<10	–	1	–	–	1
10–14	–	3	1	–	4
15–19	1	1	–	3	5
20–24	3	1	2	1	7
25–29	4	–	1	2	7
30+	2	–	1	1	4

Note: Two home helps did not answer this question.

home helps who responded to the questionnaire did personal care as well as domestic work.

Home helps receive very little training for the domestic and personal care tasks that they are required to undertake. All the respondents except two said they had done the three-day (18-hour) basic home help course. This covers the duties and responsibilities of the home help, lifting and handling clients, human needs, food and nutrition, hygiene, the causes and management of incontinence, and health and safety. The three senior home helps had all taken additional courses in social care. Two had City and Guilds 325/1, and one of these had also done an in-service course; the other senior was taking City and Guilds 325/2 at the time of completing the questionnaire. A number of the home helps and seniors informed me, when I accompanied them on client visits, that they were looking forward to the introduction of National Vocational Qualifications (NVQs), as this would permit the skills they used in their work to be recognized.

The three seniors all had guaranteed hours of work – 30 hours per week – and could work up to 39 hours per week. The basic home helps were all employed part time and had no guaranteed hours, so that the hours they worked could vary from week to week. (They were, however, entitled to paid sick leave and holidays.) The average hours per week worked by the home helps who completed the questionnaire varied between seven and over 30. Those in the urban areas worked longer hours than those employed in the more rural areas. Concern was expressed by the seniors and organizers that there was a shortage of work for the home helps in more rural areas and that fluctuation in hours was a problem for some of them. Only one home help referred to insufficient hours as a problem in responding to the questionnaire. Hours worked are summarized in Table 6.7.

The home helps were asked which of a range of domestic, social and personal care tasks they performed on a regular basis for at least one client, and in all four areas a wide range of tasks were indeed performed. They were also asked if they regularly did additional tasks for clients that were not part of their allocated duties. Twenty-four of them said they did. Among tasks which were mentioned were extra shopping (7), washing hair (3), dealing with correspondence (3), counselling/advice (3), talking to client (2), taking out bin (2), mending clothes (1), delivering Christmas cards (1), sorting out queries on bills (1), giving medication (tablets) (1), washing the dog (1), making cakes (1), washing paintwork (1), taking laundry home (1), taking to church (1), taking for walks (1), cooking (1), minor repairs (1), laying carpet (1), making cushions (1), checking if OK at weekends (1), generally caring for them (1). Twelve of these home helps said there were also additional tasks that they did occasionally for clients. The tasks mentioned were the same as those performed for some clients regularly. In addition, three who did not perform additional tasks for clients on a regular basis did so occasionally; the tasks mentioned were shopping, talking to them and calling back if they were poorly to see if they were all right.

Sixteen of the home helps said that clients asked them to do tasks that were not part of their official duties. Tasks mentioned included cleaning brass (2), scrubbing door step (2), cleaning windows (1), changing light bulbs (1), cleaning windows outside (7), filling hot water bottle (1), winding clock (1), sweeping yard (3), changing mattress cover (1), cutting toenails (1), cutting hair (1), scrubbing path (1), clearing outside drains (1), changing curtains (2), gardening (1), decorating (1), extra washing (1), washing paintwork (1), sitting with client while carer goes out (1), moving and cleaning underneath heavy furniture (1) and mending clothes (1). Twenty of the home helps said that clients telephoned them at home. In the majority of cases this was to ask them to do shopping for them. Five said the clients sometimes called for other reasons – generally because they required help, for example because they had fallen down.

All except three of the home helps had clients whose care was shared with district nurses. All of them thought that the arrangement worked well and all except one thought that the district nursing team carried out tasks for shared-care clients that home helps were unable to do. The tasks mentioned were skilled nursing tasks, except that one home help who did only domestic work and social care mentioned personal care. Ten of the home helps said that they had opportunity to liaise with the district nurse. One other home help said that there was liaison via a senior. The home helps seemed to feel that they had less opportunity to liaise with the district nurses than vice versa. Observation and information obtained from interviewing would indicate that this liaison was ad hoc and opportunistic rather than formalized. Indeed, one senior home help said that she would welcome more formal arrangements for liaising with the district nursing team about shared-care clients, for example by attending the team meetings.

The home helps already provided a wide range of domestic, social and personal care services for clients. In defining their job, most of them emphasized the caring or helping element. This was clearly reflected in their answers to a question on job title. Twenty-two of the 28 who answered this question did not feel that the title 'home help' adequately reflected the job they did. The vast majority of the suggested alternatives included 'carer' or 'caring' in the title, the two most frequently mentioned being 'community carer' and 'home carer'.

There was a very high level of job satisfaction, despite the fact that 22 said they had insufficient time to do the job as they thought it ought to be done. Fifteen of them felt they had insufficient time to chat with clients, although the home helps see providing social contact as an integral part of the job; four said they always had to rush to get the allocated tasks done; and seven said that it was impossible to get the allocated tasks done in the time allowed. Only two gave answers that suggested any degree of dissatisfaction with the job, however; both of them had taken it 'because it was convenient'.

Most of the home helps said they had joined the service because they wanted to help people and because they thought it was a job that would give them satisfaction. Typically, they wrote

I wanted to help others and do a job which was worthwhile and satisfying in my community.

I wanted to work and wanted to do something to help people, having looked into this job I felt that I would be able to do the necessary work and help people to retain their independence which I feel is very important.

A number also pointed out that their experience as carers in the domestic sphere – as mothers, wives and carers for dependent relatives – meant that they had the skills to do the work. Only five said they had become home helps because they needed a job and there had been a vacancy: 'It was a convenient job at the time'. Three of these added that the job was a satisfying and rewarding one:

When I first started it was just a job, but as time goes on you get involved and it seems so worthwhile, you feel you're doing something to help so many ill and old people.

This high level of job satisfaction and the intrinsic rewards of being a home help were clearly evidenced when the home help described their job. Many of them took the opportunity to highlight the rewarding element.

It makes me feel as though I really am needed.

Having the opportunity to work with the elderly/disabled allows me to use the many skills that one develops over the years. Tactfulness, having my own transport, communicating with people, is a rewarding challenge.

One summed it up by describing her job as 'worthwhile'. One of those who did not feel totally satisfied with the job nevertheless described it as 'a rewarding, varied job and at the same time not too badly paid either'. Another said, 'I love my job as a home carer'. Two of the three senior home helps, on the other hand, said they found the job insufficiently challenging, although they did get some job satisfaction from it. They also felt that the difference in pay between home helps and seniors was insufficient; it did not reflect the extra responsibility and paperwork they had to undertake.

Only one home help expressed a negative view of her work. In describing her job she said, 'Some people call us the Community Dogsbodies'. However, while we were accompanying home helps in two of the areas, a number of them referred to the negative stereotype that they thought home helps had – at least with some clients – and suggested that the district nurses (including auxiliaries) looked down on them because they were seen as doing dirty, menial work. One mentioned a meeting at which she had been with auxiliaries, where the auxiliaries had said that they would not take on the work home helps did because it was demeaning. It was clear that at least some of the home helps thought they were treated differently by clients because they were home helps. We were told that clients would not think of asking nurses to do extra tasks for them or ringing them at home, and our research bears this out.

Conclusions

The findings from interviews with 100 clients, observation of home helps and district nurses at work and questionnaires completed by home helps and members of the district nursing team confirm the findings of previous research. The main carers for frail elderly people, even when they are receiving domiciliary services, are co-resident relatives – mainly spouses. The main providers of domiciliary services for the frail elderly are the GPs, members of the district nursing team and the home helps. GPs and district nurses are primarily concerned with providing health care, though the nurses do also provide personal care. Nursing is one of the caring professions (Abbott and Wallace 1991), and holistic nursing stresses the need to regard patients as people. Many nurses 'train for the district' because they want to maintain direct contact with patients and do hands-on nursing. Nurses regard many personal care tasks as an integral part of patient care and something they are trained to do. (Although auxiliaries often undertake these tasks, they are seen as doing so under the supervision of a district nursing sister who takes responsibility for the care of the patient.)

As home helps have taken on more clients for whom they provide personal care, an overlap has developed in the tasks performed by the two services. In the areas where we carried out our research some district nurses were concerned that home helps were looking after clients for whom nurses should have been responsible. This concern has been exacerbated by changing views about the appropriate work for qualified (registered) nurses with the introduction of Project 2000 – the notion that qualified nurses should undertake only those tasks that require their specialized skills. At the time of this research this was combined with uncertainty about how the introduction of the Community Care legislation in 1993 was going to affect the district nursing service. There was concern that the role of the home help service would be expanded and that of the district nursing service contracted. Two key fears were expressed: that the role of nursing auxiliaries would be abandoned; and that frail elderly people who needed care from nursing staff would not be referred by the home helps.

I would suggest, however, that it was the home helps who did the actual caring, while district nurses performed mostly specialized nursing care. District nurses see themselves as experts providing specialist (expert) nursing care for patients. They work within a set of medical/nursing discourses which defined who their patients should be and the kind of care that they will provide. They tend to construe all the tasks they provide as needing training, and they often express concern that untrained home helps are carrying out tasks for certain clients for which they have no specific training. This ignores the fact that these personal care tasks are those which women, especially informal carers, are expected to carry out routinely without any training or nursing assistance. Home helps, before they are recruited to the service, have generally had many years' experience of carrying out precisely these tasks for their families.

We were told by district nurses that many clients preferred having personal care tasks performed by nurses, because people accepted help from nurses, but did not like home helps performing these tasks. However, personal care tasks are often done by auxiliaries, who are recruited from the same female labour pool as home helps and, like them, receive a minimum of formal training. The people interviewed in the three GP practices in Cornwall expressed a very high level of satisfaction with all the services provided by home helps; overall, indeed, there tended to be a higher level of satisfaction with the home helps than with the district nurses.

Perhaps this is not surprising. Our observation led us to see the home helps as caring, friendly and concerned. The district nurses, while friendly and caring, tended to be more formal and to maintain a professional distance. This was reinforced by the different ways in which clients were allocated to home helps and to district nurses. Clients were allocated to a particular home help, and they knew on which days of the week and what times of the day she would come. The timing of home help visits was negotiated with clients, taking into account their preferences and the tasks to be performed. The district nurses rotated clients and times of visit. Less attention was paid to client preferences (although these were not ignored), and clients who were to be helped to have a bath could be visited at any time during the morning. The priority in ordering clients was nursing need and operational needs; for example, diabetics had to be visited first, and in one area all patients who were to give samples of blood had to be visited early so that the samples could be back at the GP practice for collection by 11 a.m. Patients were allocated to nurses or auxiliaries in such a way that the latter travelled in any one day within a geographically limited area. This meant that the home helps were able to develop more of a relationship with clients, which was often helped by the fact that they lived in close proximity, knew the same people as the client and had a shared interest in the locale. Indeed, the home helps saw providing social contact for their clients as a central part of the job. District nurses tended to think that home helps spent too much time talking to clients and not enough getting on with the work – an attitude deriving at least in part from nurse training, where they were expected to keep busy on the wards and not spend time talking to patients (Melia

1987). This is not to say that the nurses did not talk to patients, or that they were unfriendly. Clearly, however, home helps were seen by clients as approachable and helpful. This is evidenced by the extent to which clients were prepared to ask them to do extra tasks and to telephone them in their own homes to ask for assistance.

Home helps not only do 'extras' for clients; they also work hard to carry out the tasks they have been allocated. They care about their work and their clients and take a pride in doing the work well. I suggest that home helps are not only the main providers of services for frail elderly people living on their own but also the main carers. Women are caring for women. They work hard to get the task allocation done, they work in their own time, and in general they care about their clients. There is no evidence of a 'caring community' taking on responsibility for frail elderly people living alone – the caring community does not seem to exist for these people – but the care is provided by the home help.

The home help service, in Cornwall as elsewhere, has increasingly become a service provided for frail elderly people who would otherwise be at risk of having to go into residential care. The home helps perform a range of domestic, social and personal care tasks for clients. They do so seven days a week, throughout the year. They are paid to care, but this research strongly suggests that they generally *do* care. Home helps are, generally, married working-class women who want part-time work that fits in with other domestic commitments. Although they are often portrayed as an exploited group of female workers who are paid low wages and have poor conditions of employment, in our research the post of home help was seen by those who held it as 'a good job'. The women who became home helps saw the job as satisfying work where they could use the skills they had acquired as carers for their own families, as work that fitted in with the other demands of their lives, and as comparatively well remunerated. One home help organizer told us she was dreading advertising a home help vacancy, as she knew she would be inundated with applications. Home helps think of themselves as doing the work they would do for their families; one, talking about personal care work for an elderly female client, said that she first thought of her as like her mother and did for her what she would do for her mother. It seems to me that many home helps think of clients as if they were family and that clients think of home helps as like a daughter, rather than home helps thinking of themselves as paid cleaners or care givers and clients thinking of them as domestic servants or nurses. This tends to increase the extent to which home helps think of themselves as carers and clients treat home helps as people whom they can ask to do extra tasks or call on when there is an emergency. This is reinforced by gender ideologies; women are *expected* to care, to be self-sacrificing and to be good at caring and domestic tasks.

Note

* This paper is based on data collected as part of funded research into the skills mix involved in domiciliary services for older and chronically sick or disabled people,

carried out for the Cornwall Social Services, Community Health Trust and Family Health Service Authority. The views expressed are those of the author alone. I should like to thank Gloria Lankshear, Jo Cooke and Pam Pinder, who carried out the interviews with clients.

References

Abbott, P. A. (1994) Conflict over the grey areas: Home helps and district nurses providing community care. *Journal of Gender Studies*, 3(3): 299–306.

Abbott, P. A. and Sapsford, R. J. (1993) Studying policy and practice: The use of vignettes. *Nurse Researcher*, 1(2): 81–91 (reprinted as Chapter 7 of this volume).

Abbott, P. A. and Wallace, C. (eds) (1991) *The Sociology of the Caring Professions*. London: Falmer.

Cornwall Social Services (undated) *Some Facts and Figures*. Truro: Cornwall County Council.

Lennon, J. (1991) *Cornwall: Rural Deprivation*. Truro: Cornwall Social Services.

Melia, K. (1987) *Learning and Working: The Occupational Socialisation of Nurses*. London: Tavistock.

Office of Population Censuses and Surveys (OPCS) (1986) *General Household Survey 1985*. London: HMSO.

Social Services Inspectorate (SSI) (1987) *From Home Help to Home Care*. London: DHSS.

Social Services Inspectorate (SSI) (1991) *Care Management and Assessment: Managers' Guide*. London: HMSO.

SEVEN

STUDYING POLICY AND PRACTICE: USE OF VIGNETTES

Pamela Abbott and Roger Sapsford

The research reported on in this chapter looked at the provision of domiciliary 'community care' services for people over the age of 65; the specific brief was to examine the mix of skills in the delivery of services, and a mix of methods was used, including interviews with older people and their carers, observation of practice and questionnaires to home helps, district nurses and their managers. The full results have been outlined elsewhere (Abbott 1992).

The main aim of this chapter is to outline the way in which the technique of obtaining judgements about vignettes was employed for systematic exploration of policy and practice. It is suggested that direct questioning of clients or practitioners, even coupled with observation, does not reveal the reasons or systematic patterns underlying their decisions; for this, a different kind of means is needed, and vignettes offer a good method of exploring such aspects of policy.

The vignette study

The technique of presenting 'dummy situations' in the form of brief descriptions has been widely used in social psychology, for example to study group decision-making (Kogan and Wallach 1964; Pruitt 1971) or to examine the basis of individuals' moral reasoning (Kohlberg 1969, 1976). They have also been used in both Britain and the USA for the study of professional decisions about what constitutes child abuse taken by social workers and health visitors (Giovannoni and Becerra 1979; Dingwall and Fox 1986) and to examine public attitudes to community care (West *et al.* 1984).

Their advantages for the study of how decisions are reached are that:

- while obviously artificial, they come nearer to the real situation than generalized questions about attitudes or policies because they enable us to study the decisions taken in particular cases;
- they can be varied systematically to cover a wider range of features of the situation than would be likely to crop up in most direct observation studies;
- they have the advantage of all questionnaire research in that they can be presented to a large sample, so yielding data of some generality.

During the questionnaire and observation stages of the research into the 'skills mix' employed in community care – the extent to which home helps or the district nurses, or both, were allocated to people in need of care – marked differences emerged between the practice in our three target areas; they were dissimilar, particularly, in the amount and kind of personal care undertaken by district nursing teams. The original research design was therefore extended to explore the policy and practice of a wider range of areas within the county.

All of the people responsible for the allocation of cases and their overall management throughout the county, the home help organizers and district nursing team leaders, were sent a brief questionnaire which included a set of structured vignettes – brief descriptions of 'cases' whose circumstances they might have to assess in their day to day practice. A total of 19 organizers replied, and 28 team leaders.

The vignettes, an illustrative selection of which is covered in the next section, were based loosely on 'real-life cases' encountered during the observation phase of the research, but fictionalized to an extent to preserve anonymity and to permit the systematic coverage of a wide range of situations. For each, respondents were asked to say who should mainly be responsible for each of a list of care tasks, from a list of 15 potential service-providers. Respondents were able to nominate any number of these as the appropriate source of care, separately for each task – in other words, to say whether the responsibility should be shared.

For the current analysis, responses have been clustered into:

- district nursing team and home helps;
- home helps;
- district nursing team;
- neighbours or friends;
- spouse or relatives;
- other.

The codes are pre-emptive – each respondent is entered only once, in the lowest-numbered category possible. In some tables, percentages may not add to 100 because some respondents thought that the client – and only the client – should take responsibility for a particular kind of care.

Illustrative findings

Case 1: Mr and Mrs Jones

Mr and Mrs Jones, who are in their early 70s, live in a modern bungalow about a mile from local shops and 10 miles from the nearest town. They both have occupational pensions in addition to the state's. Mrs Jones can drive, but Mr Jones, who has Parkinson's disease, has severe mobility problems and is no longer able to leave the house without professional assistance. He attends the day hospital one day a week and has regular periods of respite care. Mrs Jones has a heart condition and has had two hip replacements – both of which are now

Table 7.1 Responses to Vignette 1

Care task	Home help organizers DN+HH	DN	HH	N/F	Rel	Other
Bathing/showering						
Mr Jones	% 44	17	28	–	–	11
Helping him wash	% 11	–	89	–	–	–
Shaving him	% 6	–	88	–	6	–
Treating						
pressure areas	% 17	78	–	–	–	6
Oral hygiene	% 15	15	45	–	20	–
Getting Mr Jones						
up and dressed	% 22	–	78	–	–	–
Getting Mr Jones						
undressed	% 32	–	68	–	–	–
Shopping	% –	–	78	6	17	–
Meal preparation	% –	–	44	–	38	18
Laundry	% –	–	27	–	20	53
Light housework	% –	–	28	–	22	50

Care task	District nurse team leaders DN+HH	DN	HH	N/F	Rel	Other
Bathing/showering						
Mr Jones	% 22	48	22	–	–	8
Helping him wash	% 22	4	74	–	–	–
Shaving him	% 30	7	52	–	11	–
Treating						
pressure areas	% 26	70	4	–	–	–
Oral hygiene	% 35	23	35	–	7	–
Getting Mr Jones						
up and dressed	% 22	4	70	–	4	–
Getting Mr Jones						
undressed	% 15	4	81	–	–	–
Shopping	% –	–	79	17	4	–
Meal preparation	% –	–	74	7	11	7
Laundry	% –	–	67	4	7	22
Light housework	% –	–	64	–	18	18

In this and subsequent tables, responses are based on 19 home help organizers and 28 district nursing team leaders, except where one or two respondents failed to answer or gave an uninterpretable response.

Key
DN: District nurse   HH: Home help
N/F: Neighbour/friend   Rel: Relation

causing her problems. They moved to Cornwall on retirement and have no relatives living locally.

The results for this vignette are fairly clear-cut (Table 7.1). Both organizers and team leaders see the domestic tasks as mostly appropriate for the home helps and not at all appropriate for district nurses. Treating pressure areas is seen as mostly a district nursing task, though some organizers and team leaders see a possibility of it being shared with home helps, whereas helping Mr Jones to wash is seen as mostly a home help task, though sometimes as a shared one.

The major discrepancy comes in the category of 'bathing/showering', where team leaders are more likely to see this as appropriate for the district nurses, and organizers more likely to see it as appropriate for home helps. The other interesting points are: that housework, laundry and meal preparation are seen as tasks for which Mrs Jones should take responsibility, despite her heart condition and mobility problems, by about a fifth of the district nursing team leaders and almost as many of the home help organizers; and that a small – but not trivial – proportion of both services regard it as reasonable that neighbours should take responsibility for some social/domestic care tasks. (The 'other' category comprises the day hospital for personal care tasks, meals on wheels, and private cleaners and laundry services.)

Case 2: Mr and Mrs Smith

Mr and Mrs Smith live in council housing specifically built for disabled people. Mr Smith, who is in his mid-80s, is still fairly active. Mrs Smith, in her 60s, is confined to a wheelchair, has virtually no mobility and is registered blind. They have only state benefits.

Again, the results are fairly easy to interpret (Table 7.2). The domestic tasks – shopping, preparing and cooking meals and housework – are seen as home help specialties, though less so by home help organizers than by district nursing team leaders; the former are quite likely to suggest that these tasks should be done by a relative, usually Mr Smith.

Treating pressure areas is seen mostly as a job for the district nursing team, though more strongly so by home help organizers than by district nursing team leaders. Most of the other tasks have a tendency to be allocated to home helps, though district nursing team leaders are more likely than home help organizers to think that district nurses should be involved in personal care tasks.

Most of the team leaders and the home help organizers think both home helps and district nurses should be involved in providing care. It is interesting to note that gender seems to influence the extent to which the district nursing team leaders think that a spouse should be providing care; overall, Mr Smith was nominated for each task substantially less often than Mrs Jones.

Case 3: Mrs Johnstone

Mrs Johnstone, who is in her 70s, lives in a small bungalow about five minutes' walk from the local village store/post office. Her divorced daughter lives next door, calls in daily and gets her mother's shopping. Mrs Johnstone recently had a fall and cut her leg open; the wound is healing very slowly.

Table 7.2 Responses to Vignette 2

Care task	Home help organizers DN+HH	DN	HH	N/F	Rel	Other
Washing Mrs Smith	% 32	–	68	–	–	–
Treating pressure areas	% 16	79	–	–	–	5
Washing her hair	% 5	–	79	5	11	–
Oral hygiene	% 28	17	11	–	44	–
Getting Mrs Smith up and dressed	% 26	–	74	–	–	–
Getting Mr Smith undressed	% 6	21	57	–	16	–
Shopping	% –	–	50	–	50	–
Meal preparation	% –	–	38	6	50	6
Cooking meals	% –	–	26	6	62	6
Light housework	% –	–	58	–	42	50

Care task	District nurse team leaders DN+HH	DN	HH	N/F	Rel	Other
Washing Mrs Smith	% 41	15	44	–	–	–
Treating pressure areas	% 33	63	4	–	–	–
Washing her hair	% 17	29	50	–	–	4
Oral hygiene	% 42	29	25	–	4	–
Getting Mrs Smith up and dressed	% 22	11	67	–	–	–
Getting Mr Smith undressed	% 11	11	78	–	–	–
Shopping	% –	–	74	11	11	4
Meal preparation	% –	–	78	4	14	4
Cooking meals	% –	–	74	–	15	11
Light housework	% –	–	81	4	11	4

See Table 7.1 for key

Table 7.3 suggests a general consensus that dressing the leg wound is a nursing job (the 'other' mentioned by home help organizers is the practice nurse), and helping to have a shower is seen as a nursing job by the team leaders, but not particularly by the home help organizers. Two-thirds of the team leaders and three-quarters of the home help organizers nominated only the district nursing service for this case. Both see housework as the daughter's role.

Case 4: Mr Carter

Mr Carter, who is in his 70s, lives in a farmhouse about two miles outside a small town. He lives with his wife and unmarried son.

Table 7.3 Responses to Vignette 3

| Care task | Home help organizers | | | | | |
	DN+HH	DN	HH	N/F	Rel	Other
Dressing leg wound	% –	95	–	–	–	5
Help with having shower	% 11	22	22	–	39	6
Light housework	% –	–	17	6	77	–

| Care task | District nurse team leaders | | | | | |
	DN+HH	DN	HH	N/F	Rel	Other
Dressing leg wound	% –	100	–	–	–	–
Help with having shower	% 4	70	7	–	19	–
Light housework	% –	–	19	–	81	–

See Table 7.1 for key

Table 7.4 Responses to Vignette 4

| Care task | Home help organizers | | | | | |
	DN+HH	DN	HH	N/F	Rel	Other
Treating pressure areas	% 16	79	5	–	–	–
Washing	% 39	–	39	–	22	–
Bath	% 16	67	6	–	–	11
Getting up/dressed	% 42	–	42	–	16	–
Getting undressed/to bed	% 35	–	35	–	30	–

| Care task | District nurse team leaders | | | | | |
	DN+HH	DN	HH	N/F	Rel	Other
Treating pressure areas	% 12	80	4	–	4	–
Washing	% 40	4	26	–	26	4
Bath	% 12	57	12	–	4	15
Getting up/dressed	% 27	8	35	–	30	–
Getting undressed/to bed	% 16	4	40	–	40	–

See Table 7.1 for key

Another son and daughter-in-law live close by. Mr Carter has no feeling in the lower part of his body and is incontinent. There is a hoist for getting him in and out of bed. He attends a day centre for two days a week.

As we can see from Table 7.4, this is one case where substantial amounts of shared care are recommended; around 40 per cent of home help organizers think that dressing/undressing and washing should involve both services, and district nurses agree about the washing, while a smaller but substantial proportion are prepared to see other tasks as shared.

Over 80 per cent of home help organizers suggested some element of shared care, and around 60 per cent of the district nursing team leaders. Pressure areas and baths are seen as distinctively district nurse tasks by a substantial proportion of the sample. Personal care is also to be supplied by relatives in a greater proportion of responses than is the case in some other vignettes.

Conclusions

The practice of those who provide statutory care for older people was studied in one English county by means of questionnaires to home helps and district nurses and interviews with older people and their informal carers. These enabled us to see what services were provided and by whom – with substantial agreement between the different sources. Periods of direct observation also contributed to our understanding of practice.

Policy was studied in the first instance by a brief and relatively unstructured questionnaire to organizers and team leaders. For studying 'policy in practice' in particular cases, the periods of observation were also very useful, both revealing services which different workers provided but did not list in their questionnaires, and eliciting the rhetoric which allows particular practices under policies which might not seem on the face of it to justify or allow them.

The method which yielded the most useful information on this side of the research, however, was the vignettes to which organizers and team leaders responded. These enabled us to explore, with a larger sample of key decision-makers, the extent to which the differences we found were common across the county and between the professional groups.

The results, illustrated for four of the vignettes, suggest there is a fair amount of agreement across the two professions and within each profession about certain kinds of task – those that require specialized nursing skills and those that are clearly domestic labour. There are differences, however, in relation to personal care tasks, both between groups and within each group.

This research demonstrates that the vignette technique can contribute something to research on policy and practice which cannot be obtained by other methods. Questionnaires and interviews tell us what people say they do, and why they say they do it, but not necessarily what they actually do. Observation allows us to look at particular cases and to talk about why they are handled as they are, but with finite resources only a limited number of cases can be covered; they will inevitably be the cases that happen to be available, not necessarily the cases which would have been most informative. Vignettes can be used, as they were in this study, to cover a wider range of informants and a wider range of cases.

Further, systematic manipulation of the stimulus material would permit us to explore not just what is done, but why. In the research reported here, we were concerned only to present as wide a range of 'cases' as we had come across during the other phases of the study. In a different kind of study, however, we could have used the technique to study some aspect of policy/practice more systematically.

We could have presented vignettes which differed systematically in the gender of relatives, whether they were in employment and how far they lived from the person in need, the presence of a spouse, the age of the person in need, and even (by manipulation of the adjectives used) the character and personality of the person in need. If systematic differences in response paralleled the systematic differences in the vignettes, then something of substantive significance would have been discovered.

Perhaps the most important fact about the vignette technique, however, is that it can be used to study policy and practice without summoning up the established rhetoric which surrounds all areas of professional decision-making. There are essentially two kinds of behaviours which can be described as 'policies', and they may differ a great deal.

On the one hand, we have 'declared policy', conceived of as made by 'policy-makers'. This consists of *statements* about what should be done or about what is done, and it is properly investigated by questionnaire or interview or study of the written word. On the other hand, there is what might be called *concrete policy*, made by people we might call 'decision-makers'. Concrete policy decisions are made in the normal course of dealing with individual cases/clients, and the total of such decisions amounts to the totality of the practice under investigation. The usual tools for exploring this are the unstructured interview (but at the risk of having the description of how decisions are made contaminated by the informants' awareness of verbalized 'policy') and direct observation (a good method, but time-consuming and able to deal only with what is there to be observed). Vignettes constitute a third way of coming at 'concrete policy', and they have many potential advantages over the other two.

The drawback of the vignette technique as used here is its artificiality; respondents read summaries of cases rather than having the full data of the real-life situation, they make a limited numerical response rather than a reasoned and justified submission, and they do not have to carry out what they decide. The third of these is inherent in the method and is shared with all questionnaire/attitude research methods. The first two, however, are not inherent in the method itself. It would be possible, for example, to give a whole case-file as vignette and ask for a lengthy and reasoned written or oral report as response.

Indeed, it is possible to present 'living vignettes' and have people act out the role of client in a realistic way; Wasoff and Dobash (1992) sent research assistants in to see solicitors to act out predetermined divorce-client scenarios. In both this case and in an example giving a whole case-file as a vignette, the situation would be more like the real-life one in which decisions are made, but the price to be paid would be breadth of coverage.

Acknowledgements

Gloria Lankshear, Pam Pinder and Jo Cooke conducted the client interviews, and their hard work and commitment to the project eased the data collection phase considerably. George Giarchi provided invaluable advice at the outset of the project and warm support throughout. The research was funded out of Localities Study monies.

References

Abbott, P. (1992) *Rationalising the Skills Mix in Community Care for Disabled and Older People*. Plymouth: University of Plymouth Community Research Centre.

Dingwall, R. and Fox, S. (1986) Health visitors' and social workers' perceptions of child-care problems, in A. While (ed.) *Research in Preventive Community Nursing: Fifteen Studies in Health Visiting*. Chichester: Wiley.

Giovannoni, J. M. and Becerra, R. M. (1979) *Defining Child Abuse*. London: Collier-Macmillan.

Kogan, N. and Wallach, M. (1964) *Risk Taking: A Study of Cognition and Personality*. New York: Holt, Rinehart & Winston.

Kohlberg, L. (1969) *Stages in the Development of Moral Thought and Action*. New York: Holt, Rinehart & Winston.

Kohlberg, L. (1976) Moral stages and moralization: The cognitive-developmental approach, in T. Lickona (ed.) *Moral Development and Behavior*. New York: Holt, Rinehart & Winston.

Pruitt, D. G. (1971) Conclusions: Towards an understanding of choice shifts in group discussion. *Journal of Personality and Social Psychology*, 20: 495–510.

Wasoff, F. and Dobash, R. E. (1992) Simulated clients in 'natural' settings: Constructing a client to study professional practice. *Sociology*, 26: 333–49.

West, P., Illsley, R. and Kelmann, H. (1984) Public preference for the care of dependency groups. *Social Science and Medicine*, 18: 287–95.

CONTROLLED TRIALS AND COMPARISONS

Introduction

In this final section we look at examples of the most structured kind of research design – experiments and other designs which attempt to follow the same logic as experiments. The experiment (or controlled trial) expresses a simple logic: that if you manipulate one variable and observe that another one changes, and you can show that there is no other plausible explanation for the observed change except for the manipulation you introduced, then you may argue that your manipulation caused the change. In the simplest and clearest design there would be two identical groups of people, one of whom received a treatment while the other did not. To the extent that the groups are identical, and underwent precisely the same experiences during the research except for the presence or absence of the treatment, we may say that any observed effect is caused by the treatment. Verona Gordon's chapter in this section describes an experiment of this kind, on the treatment of depression in women. There are other kinds of design, involving multiple comparison or changes over time in the treatment of the same person or people; see for example Abbott and Sapsford (forthcoming) for details. Their underlying principles are the same, however – manipulation of an independent variable to produce changes in a dependent variable, while all extraneous influences (possible alternative explanations) are controlled.

This kind of 'scientific' research has always been popular among 'applied' researchers – researchers into policy or practice – because it impresses managers, administrators and policy-makers. It has 'the authority of science' behind it and appears to deal in 'hard facts' rather than 'subjective opinions'. It does indeed have many strengths, and it is the proper way to proceed where the topic under investigation is well understood and what is at stake is the testing of unambiguous hypotheses. Its power is sometimes overrated, however. As we said earlier, it is good for testing theory, but not good for generating theory, because it is inevitably cast in terms of preconceived concepts and is not open to discovery. It is also reductionist – it identifies 'variables' for manipulation and/or measurement – and often has difficulty relating these back to the lives and social worlds of those under investigation and the social structures within which they operate. Policy-makers have been 'educated' by the research which has been presented to them, over the years, and more 'qualitative' work is now often equally acceptable to them. Nonetheless this kind of controlled comparison remains a strong set of techniques and useful for the applied researcher.

Many classic experiments of social psychology take place in the laboratory, under controlled conditions, and are therefore open to attack on the grounds that the situation is totally unnatural; what happens in the laboratory might well not happen in ordinary life. Many others escape this criticism by taking place in a real-life setting, and this would include virtually all experimental testing of new treatment procedures and professional practices. If the subjects know that they are a part of an experiment there is an automatic alternative explanation for their behaviour – that they may be behaving as they are in order to comply with the 'rules of experiments'. (This is known as the 'Hawthorne Effect', after a famous piece of real-life research in which every change made to working conditions in a factory improved productivity – including undoing all the changes and putting things back to how they had been before the study!) It is frequent practice, therefore, to conceal the purpose of the research from the experimental subjects. Many would argue, however, that there is something unethical in manipulating subjects without their knowledge and consent, that it amounts to treating them as objects rather than as human beings.

Verona Gordon's experiment, in the first chapter in this section, passes muster in this respect; her subjects knew perfectly well what was going on. It is also worth noting that her experiment does no harm to subjects and puts no one at risk of harm or distress – something which cannot be said for all. She even avoids the charge very often levelled at controlled trials in therapy or education, that it is immoral to withhold treatment from a control group just for the sake of the experimental design. With limited resources she could handle only a relatively small number of clients in her therapy groups, and she had a large number of applicants, so she did not so much withhold treatment from the control group as capitalize on the fact that she could not deal with everyone who applied. Thus we may put her study forward as a good example of this kind of research. However, we should note that the ethical problems of experimentation are considerable; experimental designs give rise to even more misgivings and questions that need answering than other kinds of research.

Often true experiments are impossible even in principle. The quasi-experimental comparison is logically weaker than the true experiment, and more research may be needed before we can put a sensible interpretation on the results. Here we have a comparison of groups, with one receiving a treatment and others acting as 'controls', or two groups contrasted as different 'values' of a treatment variable, but the groups are naturally occurring and allocation to them is not under the control of the 'experimenter'. We may contrast men's and women's attitudes, for example, and wish to conclude something about differences between the genders, but men and women embedded in their social situations differ substantially in ways which go beyond the mere fact of gender, so it is more difficult to show that gender and not some other factor is responsible for the differences. In the Abbott paper on heart-disease research (Chapter 5) which you read in the last section, for example, a comparison is to be made between a group who travel for surgery and a group able to have surgery nearer to home, a structure which mimics the logic of the experiment. Cases are not randomly allocated to the two groups, however; they are 'naturally occurring'. This means that they may differ from each other in any number of ways, not just in whether they have to travel for surgery, so it will be difficult to demonstrate that the fact of travelling and only that fact lies at the heart of any differences.

The Doll and Hill paper reproduced as Chapter 9 is a famous example of this kind of quasi-experimental comparison and serves to illustrate the ways in which researchers may try to circumvent the limitations of the style. The heart of the paper is a comparison of smokers, former smokers who had given up and doctors who had never smoked. The main result is that those who had never smoked were substantially less likely to die than smokers during the three years following the completion of the questionnaire, and heavy smokers were more likely to die than lighter smokers. We may not safely conclude from these figures that smoking is responsible for mortality, however, until we have eliminated other possible explanations by statistical analysis (a process called *statistical control*). Two obvious possible explanations are controlled by the design; it is not the case that the differences in mortality are explained by differences in occupation or social class, because the respondents were all doctors. In this paper Doll and Hill control by statistical means for the effect of age in two ways – (1) by showing that there is no systematic relationship between amount smoked and age, and (2) by calculating an 'expected deaths' figure taking the ages of each group into account – and they show that age alone is not the explanation of the mortality. In other papers they have controlled for other possible explanations; the full research programme is outlined in Abbott and Sapsford (forthcoming).

Frequently quasi-experimental comparison is used where the true experiment is not impossible in principle, but totally unethical in practice, and the Doll and Hill paper is of this kind. It would be possible in principle to pay a group of randomly selected people to smoke heavily, or lightly, or not at all, and to note the mortality among them over the years, but this would be quite unethical if one supposed that there were any kind of connection with mortality rates. What Doll and Hill have to do, therefore, is to compare people who have inflicted this treatment on themselves and note the outcome.

The final chapter in this section also uses the comparison of existing groups to cast light on a common supposition – that Black and Asian people are discriminated against in the labour market. Looking at the occupations of women, it shows that all women suffer discrimination in the labour market, and some Black women suffer more discrimination that White women, but that there are Black and Asian groups which actually do better than White women in terms of grade of employment. A point to note about this paper is that researchers do not always have to collect their own data. Chapter 10 uses statistics from the Census and is an example of the kind of research that anyone can do using data available in major public or academic libraries, without the expense in time and money of collecting data first-hand.

Reference

Abbott, P. and Sapsford, R. (forthcoming) *Research Methods for Nurses and the Caring Professions*, 2nd edn. Buckingham: Open University Press.

TREATMENT OF DEPRESSED WOMEN BY NURSES IN BRITAIN

Verona Gordon

Introduction

Depression ranks as one of the major health problems of women today. Although prominent researchers Weissman and Klerman (1977) reported that twice as many women are depressed as men around the world, few research studies have been published on the development and utilization of treatment approaches to meet the needs of this population. The widespread growth in the number of American females of all ages suffering from depression is alarming (Guttentag *et al.* 1980). Depressed women have increased medical costs due to their repeated visits to physicians for psychosomatic complaints, chemical dependency, unnecessary gynaecological surgery, and their high psychiatric hospitalizations. Women seek counselling, however, there have been few convincing research studies on the effectiveness of traditional psychotherapies (Fiske *et al.* 1970). Due to the rising high cost of health care, treatment approaches in mental health must be efficacious, safe and cost-effective (Parloff 1980). Accelerating societal change is having an impact on women. The challenges to traditional values, roles, and expectations are a source of concern to women and generate emotional responses. Depression is one such emotional response that has been found to be a significant problem among women. Prevention of depression among this segment of society requires an understanding of women's perceptions of, and concerns about, their life situations. Women have high potential to learn, strong interest in growing, great influence over their families, and much to give others.

The purpose of this chapter is to provide more information about the phenomenon of depression in women and to describe a nurse group intervention designed by the author to alleviate depression in women ...

Review of the literature

Forty million Americans suffer from depression today and two-thirds of these people are women (Hirschfield 1980). Eminent researchers

(Dohrenwend 1973; van Keep and Prill 1975; Tucker 1977; Notman 1979) identified stressors occurring in women's daily lives which stem from personal, family, social, and cultural demands upon them. These result in feelings of frustration, inadequacy, and low self-esteem.

Problems facing women as they age in America include marital conflicts (Cherlin 1981), divorce (Gordon 1979), loss of attractiveness (Scarf 1980), conflicts at work (Powell 1977; Shields 1980), career disruptions due to husband's job change (Weissman *et al.* 1973), hysterectomy surgery (Raphael 1976; Editorial 1979; Martin *et al.* 1980), 'empty-nest' syndrome (Bart 1971; Radloff 1975), menopause (Neugarten *et al.* 1963), widowhood (Lopata 1971), declining physical health (Wittenborn and Buhler 1979), and care of elderly parents (Stevenson 1977). These factors may result in feelings of loneliness and isolation (Gordon 1982). (There is concern in America in respect to woman's influential role in her family and that she has the longest life expectancy, 78 years versus males' 70 years, and earns over half of the nation's income).

Psychological explanations

There may be three aetiological explanations for these escalating rates of depression in American women as described by theories of:

1 Lewinsohn's behavioural model.
2 Seligman's learned helplessness model.
3 Beck's cognitive model.

From the behavioural viewpoint depression occurs when a women does not perceive positive reinforcement in her daily life (Lewinsohn *et al.* 1982). The highest rate of depression in American females occurs between the ages of 25 and 44 years, probably their response to their own high expectations of work, marriage or having children. Belle (1982) found low-income single mothers most vulnerable to depression and that the rate of psychiatric treatment of their children was high. Most women working full-time earn 59 per cent less than male full-time workers for doing the same job (Barrett 1979). Eighty per cent of all women working in America tend to work in demanding 'service' jobs (factory work, cleaning, clerical, bank tellers, sales) which are low in pay and prestige (National Commission on Working Women 1979). Women who are employed find social–financial inequality, sex-role stereotyping, and negative prejudice, which result in reduced self-fulfilment and career options (Clayton *et al.* 1980; Carmen *et al.* 1981).

Unemployed, married women consistently report frustration with their roles (Neuberry *et al.* 1979). Housewives have few sources of gratification (Thurnher 1976; Radloff and Rae 1979): their work is relatively invisible and given little value or prestige. The absence of intimate supportive relationships with husband or children increases the risk of depression (Brown *et al.* 1975; Miller 1976). The fact that depression is more common among married, divorced or separated women than men is well documented (Radloff 1975). Gove (1972) reported that the strain of the marriage role is a causal factor of the higher rate of depression among women. The divorce rate in the United States has increased 96 per cent in the last decade and 50 per cent of all future marriages are predicted to end in divorce (*Los Angeles Times* 1980). The stress of divorce is felt more by women than by men due to women's lack of money, poor living conditions, and lack of job skills (Maykowsky 1980). Due to present national economy, there are a growing number of women staying in loveless, empty, and abusive marriages (Kaslow 1982). Pilisuk and Froland (1978) write that depression in women will continue to increase with the high mobility (extended families living thousands of miles apart), small family size, and high divorce rates.

In studies by Wood and Duffy (1966), Curlee (1969) and McLachlan *et al.* (1976), the middle-aged married housewife, not working outside her home, was found to be a higher consumer of alcohol in attempting to escape her isolation and loneliness.

Seligman's (1975) theory of learned helplessness exemplifies women's hopeless attitude which results in depression, withdrawal, and lack of motivation. There is growing awareness of the powerlessness of women in our male-dominated society, where women do not perceive that they have control over situations or that their actions bring rewards or recognition (Guttentag *et al.* 1980; LeDray and Chaignot 1980; Schaef 1981). Belle's (1982) work with poor single mothers is a powerful documentation of their helplessness fighting an indifferent government system. Studies by Chodoff (1972) and Goldberg (1973) report of depressed women with 'helpless' characteristics, and are supported by Radloff and Monroe (1978), Notman *et al.* (1978) and Kivett (1979).

Miller (1976) states that women have been relegated to nurturing tasks and may be forced to decide between either personal growth or development of an intimate relationship with men. The problem of wife-battering has increasingly been brought to the attention of the American public. Claerhout *et al.* (1982) state that violence occurs in 35–50 per cent of all marital relationships and that in part cultural attitudes explain the occurrence. While men are taught to be aggressive and independent, women often assume dependent and submissive roles in marital relationships. Walker (1979) suggests that these victims of domestic violence typically have low self-esteem, chronic anxiety, learned helplessness, denial, shame, guilt and psychosomatic complaints. Many women are withdrawn, depressed, and use denial to alleviate high tension levels. Johnson (1979) states that these dependent women tend to be high suicide risks.

Depression is also theorized to result from an individual's own misinterpretation of losses and life events. That depressed women tend to see themselves and the world around them in a negative manner is consistent with Beck's (1978) cognitive theory. For example, their adjustment to aging in the American youth-oriented society, where aging is not accepted (Chenitz 1979) and where negative stereotyping of aging abounds (Emery 1981). Women's attitudes toward themselves reveal low self-esteem and fears of failure (Horney 1967; Bardwick 1978), passivity and dependency (Kagan and Moss 1971; Cooperstock 1979), and a tendency to be self-critical (Lowenthal and Chiriboga 1972). All these symptoms are common to the syndrome of subclinical depression (Beck *et al.* 1979).

Treatment and prevention

There are two concerns that remain with treatment and prevention issues. One is that traditional treatment approaches by male therapists perpetuate the passivity and negative self-image of women (Weissman and Klerman 1977). The other is that while there are numerous programmes to treat depression, treatment usually begins after the depression has reached a serious level. This lack of early identification and intervention does not support nursing's commitment to prevention and health maintenance. Regarding the sex-role stereotyping, Broverman *et al.* (1970) concluded that professional therapists have described women clients as dependent, submissive, highly emotional, and less able to make important decisions than men. Brown and Hellinger (1975) found female therapists to have more understanding attitudes toward women patients. Kjervik and Palta (1978) identified the psychiatric nurse as the professional therapist who was least likely to hold stereotypic attitudes toward women.

Rationale for a nurse-facilitated group intervention

The apparent centrality of psychosocial factors to depression in women suggests that much might be done through early identification and treatment of symptoms through psychotherapeutic intervention. Once these women have been identified in urban and rural areas, growth-support groups can be established. At minimal expense these groups may provide the support necessary to develop and establish successful coping strategies for women while preventing more serious depression (Gordon and LeDray 1985).

A group approach can be far superior to individual treatment for women in that it allows contact with peers who are likely to be dealing with some of the same role conflicts (Maykowsky 1980). Coping strategies can be tested and shared within the supportive, safe environment of a group. These groups have been recognized as especially important in helping to lower the acknowledged sense of helplessness, powerlessness, and isolation of women living in communities (Davis 1977). In 1981 van Servellen and Dull identified group therapy as an effective medium to promote positive change in self-esteem of depressed women. Dinnauer *et al.* (1981) emphasize the strength of groups as providing an important structure for women's social learning. Gallese and Treuting (1981) state that a women's group 'can be a lifesaver' for women feeling overwhelming stress, such as rape victims. The value of these groups goes far beyond their original purpose and provides the individuals with a sense of community (Back and Taylor 1976).

Current literature has supported the professional nurse (minimum: baccalaureate prepared) as a facilitator of women's support groups. Loomis (1979) expected these nurses would function well as group leaders with their preparation in group dynamics and communication skills. Professional nurses (of whom 97.2 per cent in America are women) are the logical primary therapeutic change-agents in facilitating effective women's groups for the following reasons.

1 They are traditionally accepted by women as trusted, caring, and helpful health professionals.

2 Academically prepared, they understand both the physiological and psychological aspects of women.

3 They appreciate the women's significant influence and role within the family system.

4 They empathize with, rather than stereotype, the women's current problems within society.

5 They serve as a positive role model for women (Gordon 1982).

Braillier (1980) stresses the need for holistic health practice in the expanding role of the professional nurse. She feels nurses are 'ideal' resources to practise the holistic health approach since they deal with mind–body–spiritual aspects with relative ease. Professional nurses are committed to health maintenance and prevention. The efficacy for involving the client as an active participant in this emerging holistic health movement across America has been stated by Tubesing *et al.* (1977).

Description of 1983 study of depressed women in Great Britain

. . .

Aim of study

The purpose of the study was to evaluate the effectiveness of a nurse-facilitated group intervention in the alleviation of depression in women of Great Britain

The samples

Twenty women, 40–60 years of age, were selected for the study. These subjects had been recruited though a public service radio broadcast (BBC airwaves) seeking depressed women as participants. Preliminary screening took place during the eight-minute early morning public announcement by Gordon that in order for women to be eligible for the study they needed to be 40–60 years of age, they must speak English, and they should not presently be seeing a counsellor or psychiatrist. There was an overwhelming response to the broadcast from hundreds of women not only living in England but in areas as widespread as Wales, Belgium, Scotland, and France. The University of London's phone lines were flooded with calls, confirming the author's belief that depression in women is extensive. Over 200 women came to Chelsea College to meetings giving information about the study. Six meetings were scheduled at various hours of the week (i.e. Tuesdays 10 a.m., 3 p.m. and 7 p.m.; Fridays 10 a.m., 3 p.m. and 7 p.m.) to fit the plans of mothers and working women. Most women were working and came to the 7 p.m. meetings. Gordon (principal investigator) met the women in a large classroom where introductions were made and an overview of the study was given. Many women aged

20–30 years came to learn about the study and were disappointed that they were unable to participate until further group experiences were available. They shared feelings of depression. All interested women ($n = 119$) who met the criteria were assigned a code number, filled out a demographic questionnaire, signed a consent form, and were given two additional tests to further help the investigator screen these volunteers. The Beck Depression Inventory (Beck 1978) and the SCL-90-R (Derogatis 1976) were administered. Eighty-one women who scored 14–26 on the Beck test, indicating they were mildly to moderately depressed and who were also within 'normal limits' on the SCL-90-R (therefore were not psychotic, psychopathic or suicidal) were eligible to be group members. However, the study could only include 20 women, therefore the need for random selection was indicated. All (81) code numbers were placed in a box and the first 10 numbers drawn out by a visiting psychologist were assigned to the control group, the second 10 code numbers pulled out by this same psychologist were assigned to the experimental group. The following week all women who came to the information meeting were informed by letter of their inclusion or exclusion in the study. Eight women who showed no depression on the Beck's test were thanked but dismissed. Thirty women who showed severe depression on the Beck's test were given information about professional resource help. Of these 30 women, six were found to be most severely depressed and the investigator informed them by telephone that their initial tests indicated that they were very depressed. The women confirmed these test results and were co-operative about seeing their general practitioner the next day. All reported back to Gordon that they had been given medication and were under the direct supervision of their physicians.

Of the 20 selected subjects, all women were White, upper middle-class, with a mean age of 51 years. Eight women were married and had children, while one was divorced, five were separated, four were single, and two were widowed. Twelve women were working, one was unemployed, while seven were homemakers. Demographic differences in the experimental and control groups appeared incidental regarding age, marital status, working full-time or part-time.

Instruments used in the study

For selection of subjects

Beck Depression Inventory
This inventory (Beck 1978) is a 21-item, self-report measure (range = 0–63) used to measure level of depression. The internal consistency and validity of this widely used instrument has been well documented (Beck and Beamesderfer 1974; Shaw 1977). The score of 14–22 is in the mild–moderate depressed range and was chosen to obtain a sample of subjects.

Test–retest stability (97 cases) over a one-week interval was high ($r = 0.86$ to 0.93) and the measure appears sensitive to spontaneous or treatment related change (Beck 1972). There was a correlation coefficient of 0.75 between the Beck test and Hamilton Rating Scale (Schwab *et al.*

1967). The instrument was highly effective in discriminating between depression and anxiety (Beck 1978).

The SCL-90-R Inventory

This inventory (Derogatis 1976) is a 90-item self-report measure (norm T score = 50, SC = 10) used to screen for pathology and suicide risk. Designed to reflect nine psychological symptoms (obsessive–compulsive, somatization, paranoid ideation, psychoticism, depression, anxiety, hostility, phobic anxiety and interpersonal sensitivity) seen in psychiatric patients. Measures of internal consistency were obtained from 219 hospitalized volunteers. Alpha coefficients ranged from 0.77 to 0.90 for the dimension scores. Test–retest coefficient for 94 psychiatric outpatients (over a one-week interval) ranged from 0.80 to 0.90 The SCL-90-R correlated high 0.88 with the Minnesota Multiphasic Personality Inventory. With the Middlesex Hospital Questionnaire, six symptom dimensions were contrasted, aggregate score correlation was 0.92 (Derogatis 1976). The SCL-90-R was chosen as the one-time assessment measure for these depressed women because of the need to eliminate from the study those who did show symptoms of psychosis, psychopathology and suicide risk

Pre- and post-test (Comparison of control–experimental groups)

Coopersmith's Self-esteem Inventory

This inventory (Ryden 1978) is a 58-item self-report used to measure self-esteem in adult subjects. The test was found to have a test–retest reliability of 0.80 for 32 women over periods of 6–58 weeks. The high level of stability over a period of 58 weeks reinforces the idea that the evaluative aspect of one's concept of self, as reflected in self-report, has a considerable degree of consistency over time. Because self-esteem may be related to a person's depression, Ryden's modification of the Coopersmith's Self esteem Inventory was chosen to measure the subject's self-esteem.

The Social Adjustment Self-report

The SAS (Weissman and Paykel 1974) is a 42-item instrument that measures overall social adjustment as well as performance in six major areas of functioning: work, family, social roles, etc. Self-report results based on 76 depressed out-patients were comparable to those obtained from relatives as well as by a rater who interviewed the patient directly. This measure was validated using depressed out-patients and is capable of discriminating between recovered patients and those in acute stages of illness. Validity data show that the instrument correlates highly with independent ratings of overall social adjustment made by mental health professionals ($r = 0.72$) and by significant others ($r = 0.74$). The SAS is also sensitive to change and yields significant differences in scores before and after treatment (Bothwell and Weissman 1977).

Life Experience Survey

The purpose of the LES (Sarason et al. 1978) is to measure life changes. Advantages of this 57-item measure are that it allows for separation of

positive and negative life experiences as well as individualized ratings of
the impact of events. Test–retest reliability (at 5–6 weeks) is 0.56–0.88.
Correlations with social desirability were 0.05 to 0.01 showing good
discriminative validity. Correlations with illness, although low (0.3–0.4),
are consistent with other stress measures. The LES was chosen for this
study to help identify and measure stress areas of women subjects.

The Young Loneliness Inventory
The YLS (Young 1981) is a 19-item self-report inventory used to diagnose
the severity of recent loneliness. Various test items assess the client's
relationship with friends and close family members during a given period
of time, by rating on a scale of 0 (low) to 3 (high) the *frequency, disclosure,
caring* and *physical intimacy* they experienced in each relationship. Young
establishes cutting scores as 8–9 (normal), 10–18 (mild), 19–29 (moderate
to severe), 30 (high), and 50 (as a very high degree of loneliness). The YLS
has been tested for reliability and validity with both out-patient, college,
and university populations. In assessing reliability, measures of consistency were obtained with these populations. Alpha coefficients ranged
from 0.78 in the college to 80 in the university, to 0.84 in the mood
clinic, and were considered reasonably high.

Beck Depression Inventory – 'significant other' form
The BDI has been adapted for completion by significant other(s) of the
identified patient (Hollon 1980). All 21 items from the original inventory
have been left intact other than being worded in the third person, and
scoring principles are identical to those for the self-report form. While
little validity data are yet available for the 'significant other' form of the
BDI, initial information indicated that test provides a reasonably satisfactory
means of assessing depression.

Pre-post-testing

All subjects (*n* = 20) were given the five self-report tests described
(Coopersmith's Self-esteem, Weissman's Social Adjustment Scale, Young's
Loneliness Scale, Sarason's Life Experience Survey and the Beck Depression test filled out by a 'significant other') before the first group session
started and after the fourteenth group session was over. Test scores from
the control group and experimental groups were compared and changes
in levels of depression, self-esteem and loneliness, etc. were analysed.

Procedure

Group sessions

After meeting screening criteria (over radio and at the information meeting) subjects were randomly assigned to either the experimental (treatment, *n* = 10) or control (no-treatment, *n* = 10) condition. The treatment
consisted of 14 weekly (two-hour) group sessions led by two professional
nurses with group experience (one psychiatric nurse expert came highly
recommended from Maudsley Hospital, London, one nurse with a master's

degree in psychiatric nursing came from the USA). These nurses were briefly orientated on the structured group intervention, which utilized a holistic health approach with concepts from the cognitive–behaviour–affective models. The nurse facilitators were provided with a training manual the contents of which included group dynamics, reinforcement theory, and evaluation of group process. Lecture content with specific objectives and discussion questions for each of the 14 group sessions were also included in the training manual.

The experimental group

Women in the experimental group chose to meet at 7–9 p.m. on Monday evenings in a comfortable room at Chelsea College (May–August 1983). The setting was located in a convenient, safe area of London. Some women came by car but most of them came by bus or subway trains.

During the first two sessions each woman was given equal time to 'tell her story'. After that second session repeated recounting of problems was not encouraged. The structure of group sessions devoted the first hour to lecture, education, and discussion, while the second hour was spent in activities related to the session topic. Each woman was provided with a workbook and was expected to come to the group sessions with assigned homework completed. Weekly topics included content found in the women's workbook: goal setting, signs and symptoms of depression, cognitions and feelings, self-worth, building relationships, communication skills, assertiveness, conflict management and decision-making, stress, relaxation, exercise, nutrition, menstruation/menopause and strength building.

All group sessions were tape-recorded for the first three sessions but this was discontinued due to inability to hear voices clearly. The women were delighted to see the tape-recorder removed.

The control group

Women assigned to the control condition received no intervention between pre- and post-testing. At the first information meeting they had been asked to refrain from joining other therapy groups or seeking counselling while the study was going on unless necessary. Eight women in the control condition expressed a desire to be included in later group sessions if others were to be offered.

Results

Analysis of the data

There were no significant mean pre-treatment differences between the two treatment conditions on any of the five self-report tests, indicating that the randomization procedure was successful.

Because estimation of 'raw change' scores as measures of effectiveness of a treatment is subject to difficulties in interpretation (Cronbach and

Furby 1970), the Cohen and Cohen (1975) procedure for analysis of partial variance was used to assess the effectiveness of the treatment programme.

Statistically significant post-test differences between the control and treatment groups were demonstrated for depression, self-esteem and hopelessness. Over 35 per cent of the variance in post-test depression scores was linearly accounted for by the pre-test depression scores. Once the effects of the pre-test were removed, the treatment condition accounted for approximately 40.4 per cent of the variance in regressed change in depression from pre-test to post-test $(F = (1,17) = 11.52, p < 0.025)$. Adjustments for unreliability of the depression measure using a reliability estimate of 0.86 also resulted in significant differences between the control and treatment groups $(F = (1,17) = 13.41, p < 0.005)$. This difference represented almost one full standard deviation difference in post-test depression scores for the two groups and a classification difference from 'mild–moderate' to 'mild' on Beck's inventory.

Statistically significant improvement in scores on Coopersmith's Self-esteem Inventory was also demonstrated for subjects in the treatment condition in comparison to those in the control group. While 54 per cent of the variance in post-test self-esteem scores could be linearly accounted for by pre-test levels of self-esteem, approximately 58.8 per cent of the variance in regressed change from pre-test to post-test was accounted for by treatment condition $(F = (1,17) = 24.23, p < 0.001)$. Adjustments for unreliability of the self-esteem measure using 0.80 as an estimate of reliability yielded even higher statistically significant results $(F = (1,17) = 56.92, p < 0.001)$. Mean post-test scores adjusted for unreliability and pre-test performance were 63.78 for the treatment group and 48.12 for the control group. Again, the treatment group was almost one full standard deviation above the control group in post-test self-esteem level.

Feelings of hopelessness were also significantly reduced between pre-test and post-test for the treatment subjects, whereas there was an increase in these feelings for the control group over the same period. Over 20 per cent of the variance in post-test hopelessness scores was accounted for by pre-test feelings of hopelessness and 45.2 per cent of the variance in regressed change in hopelessness scores was accounted for by the treatment manipulation $(F = (1,17) = 14.01, p < 0.005)$. No direct reliability estimates for the Beck Hopelessness Scale were available so a reliability of 0.80 was assumed. Adjustments to the analysis based upon this level of reliability resulted in higher levels of statistical significance $(F = (1,17) = 20.81, p < 0.001)$. Subjects in the treatment group $(X = 5.76)$ scored over six units below the subjects in the control group $(X = 11.82)$. This difference between treatment and control groups represented over one standard deviation difference in performance.

Similar analyses were applied to the remaining dependent measures. No statistically significant differences between control and treatment groups on the post-test measures for loneliness, depression as rated by a significant other, social adjustment or anxiety level were observed. Perhaps the 14-week time interval for the study was not a sufficient time period to observe significant changes on these variables. Also, the significant other form of the Beck Depression Inventory is not as valid as the self-report form and, generally, measures of depression by significant others tend to underestimate self-report measures of depression. Both of these could have affected the results of the study.

The findings suggest that nurse-facilitated groups do provide a therapeutic value to moderately depressed women. The 14-week time interval was sufficient to demonstrate improvement in subjects' feelings of self-esteem and reduction in their feelings of depression and hopelessness. It seems reasonable that improvement in a woman's feelings of self-esteem and self-concept could potentially stress other aspects of her life as she learned to cope with her new sense of being and with others in her life. Also, it is possible that others, especially significant others in her life, must also learn to adapt to a woman with higher feelings of self-esteem. Perhaps this accounts for the lack of significant change in the feelings of loneliness, social adjustment, and anxiety observed in this study. Further studies should investigate this possibility.

Condensed data in notebooks

Observation notes were carefully written by both nurse group-facilitators after each session. The date, the number of members present, and the reactions of members relating to lateness or absence of peers were recorded in notebooks. Individual verbal/non-verbal behaviour was described, as well as indications of group stages, themes, and cohesiveness observed. The group met during summer 1983.

The wealth of information emerging from the content of the notebooks was too great to be included in this single chapter, however specific data observed during each session is described. Names have been changed for confidentiality.

Session 1

All women arrived on time, except Diane who had 'forgotten' about a previous engagement. All members were well dressed, neat. They looked like serious business women as introductions were made. Everyone was polite and interested. During the nurse's explanation of expectations for group leaders and members, rules of confidentiality, etc. most women sat with folded arms and guarded facial expressions. After tea and coffee, the members seemed to feel more relaxed with the two nurses gently inviting more trust. Many questions indicating anxiety about their own expectations of the group sessions arose. There was denial of feelings, i.e. 'Well, there really isn't much to talk about,' or 'Oh, I couldn't talk about anger because I have never felt it.' Two women felt there was danger in becoming 'too introspective'. Several shared their loathing of lies. Themes: mistrust, anger, sadness, and some wonder of 'how "things" at home can really change'.

Session 2

All women were punctual. With little hesitation they went into talking about their life problems. There were 'moving' moments as the women revealed their suffering and how they had suppressed a lot of their own feelings for the 'good of the family'. Support for each other was evident, i.e. 'Yes, I know what you mean, I felt that pain too when my children left home.' Women appeared more positive, they said they looked forward to coming to the group, i.e. 'It's good that there are others we can talk to.' Themes: marriage vs career, the freedom and the frustrations of living alone. Stages: trust, some cohesiveness, i.e. use of 'we' instead of 'me'.

Session 3

Nearly everyone was talking at once. Much discussion, 'advice-giving'. The group felt very charged and intense, with great sharing of deep losses, personal failures in life. Several spoke of painful separation from family when sent to boarding schools. Facilitators felt exhausted after the session and were concerned that 'too much was shared too early'.

Session 4

The group was dominated by Lisa who spent a great deal of time on frivolous events in her life; there was much chit-chat and unheeded advice-giving. Nurse-facilitators found themselves irritated that the group was not 'moving', that there seemed to be a conscious avoidance of sharing deep feelings . . . perhaps too painful from the last session. Nurses did intervene, taking control of the storytelling and the women grew thoughtful. Themes: loneliness, feelings of low self-worth, loss of male companionship.

Session 5

Three members were absent. The group appeared quiet, serious, more of a 'working' group. More intimacy emerged, e.g. how they felt powerless in marital relationships with their husbands who 'did what they wanted'. Tremendous denial of their anger toward others. They tended to blame themselves that their children did not meet their expectations, that they were concerned and hurt how their children reacted to relatives, friends. Stage: intimacy.

Session 6

Again much 'advice-giving' (how to lose weight, etc.) was apparent, and facilitators needed to get the group back to talking about the assigned homework on discussing feelings. It was a very productive session with much clarification of negative and positive feelings, of how 'should', 'ought', 'must' thinking causes their feelings of hopelessness. One woman shared how hard it was being the 'other' woman in a relationship and received support and understanding.

Session 7

Homework assignment related to learning how difficult it was to learn how to be assertive. They said they were 'brought up' to be nice, lovely ladies and it was easier to remain passive. They found it most difficult to be aggressive and nearly impossible to be assertive. Some 'pairing off' by group members, some non-direct hostility toward a domineering member.

Session 8

'Entire group came looking very pretty tonight', wrote one nurse-facilitator. The women initiated discussion on the value of the group. One woman had been turned down twice that week for jobs, but had looked forward to coming to the group for support. Much sincere feedback and support was evident. Karen said she could take what she learned in each group session and apply it daily. Facilitators felt sad and shared these feelings with the group: many women had said that this group was the 'only' place they felt they could speak freely and easily. Stage: conesiveness, group running itself.

Session 9

Vera was leaving the group for a new job in southeast Asia. Fears and anxieties were expressed by Vera. All members told her they were happy for her, sad for themselves, and a bit envious of her new adventure. She thanked them for their caring and was taking her Women's Workbook with her. Again when advice was given to various members Elaine expressed frustration that members weren't allowing self-decision-making. Reactions were highly defended and difficult. Facilitators felt the group seemed blocked and permitted power struggles.

Session 10

No absences. Group members seemed much more serious, using workbooks, reflecting more on their own reactions to daily stress. Both nurses wrote: 'These women are bright, of high intelligence, and gain insight with relative ease.' Lisa appears to have learned constructive ways of dealing with conflicts regarding her employer. More women said they had more energy and more interest in life.

Session 11

Much discussion on feelings of failure as mothers. Expressions of anger, guilt. There was beginning talk about how sad it was that the group would soon come to an end. Reflections about Vera separating from them to go to Asia brought out an atmosphere of sombre mellowness. Peggy shared for the first time that she was chemically dependent. The group was surprised at this, but supported her for continuing to come to group and work on her low self-esteem. Women went on to discuss the problem of being divorced and having no job skills. (This is a similar problem of middle-aged women in the United States.)

Session 12

Much talk of guilt when they say 'no' to doing favours for others and what to do about that guilt. Some pressure on facilitators to come up with answers. Many spoke of resistance to physical exercise. Some insight on how they resist change throughout their lives and it brings them depression. 'It is hard to change our habits.' Good discussion on the fears of taking risks to change. Definite cohesiveness between members . . . women see the facilitators as members.

Session 13

Discussion of menstruation and menopause evoked feelings of the loss of childbearing ability for some members. Support was given to each other. Others spoke of the pains of motherhood. One shared how much the group had helped her to see her children more objectively, to give them freedom to be adults, and be more accepting of her son and his 'unconventional' behaviour. She said she felt much happier in herself and that she couldn't have achieved that without help of the group. Afterwards group facilitators felt frustrated because there had not been enough time to discuss the sexual conflicts alluded to by several members.

Session 14

The last group centred on sexuality: both strategies for building positive and intimate sexual relationships, as well as sources for sexual conflict were discussed. Some women described sexual conflicts with their lovers or husbands, others explained their relationships lacked all sexual intimacy. It was interesting to observe how relaxed most of the women were discussing such personal problems. The last half hour of this session was used for group evaluation and feedback. The women felt sad that it was their last group because they felt that they had learned to trust and confide in each other. One member said she had never considered that the group would end. There was a consensus of opinion by all members and facilitators that the number of group meetings should be expanded to at least 20 sessions, so that the women would have more time to learn and test the coping skills they needed in meeting their daily problems. Facilitators felt more time was needed for termination. All the women described the groups as helpful, insightful, and supportive. They hoped to remain in touch with each other and there was an exchange of addresses. The women also gave cards and gifts to the nurses, who felt it was a wonderful experience for them. All left with much handshaking, some hugging, and tear-filled eyes.

Summary and implications for nursing

The widespread incidence of depression in women is identified as a major health problem in the world today. Prominent researchers report that women are twice as likely as men to suffer from depression. This chapter provides documentation of the stress factors that occur in women's daily lives which stem from social, family, and cultural demands on them. Women are still regarded as 'second-class' citizens with society's expectation that they are caretakers of men and children first while their own potential for self-actualization is disregarded. A consequence of this lack of recognition decreases women's self-fulfilment and self-worth. Women are the most underutilized talent in the world. Their sensitivity, creativeness, management skills, and enduring strength in crisis is taken for granted and undervalued. As a result they have feelings of frustration, inadequacy, and low self-esteem. Close relationships with significant others are of utmost importance to women. It is around attachment issues, more than any other sorts of issues, that depressive episodes in women tend to emerge. Women invest highly in intimate relationships with men and their children and to fail in those relationships, or to have them end becomes equated with failing in everything. Conflicts with husbands, children, in-laws, and lovers are cited by women as principal causes for their depression. Depressed women in America have increased medical costs due to their repeated visits to physicians for psychosomatic complaints, chemical dependency, unnecessary gynaecological surgery, and high admissions to psychiatric hospital units. Due to the rising cost of health care, treatment approaches need to be efficacious, safe and cost-effective . . .

Preliminary studies were conducted in the United States with 38 women (40–60 years of age) as subjects. The purpose of the studies was to evaluate the effectiveness of a group intervention facilitated by professional nurses in alleviating depression in women. Pre-post-testing revealed that women who attended the structured group sessions showed a significant reduction in depression and a significant increase in self-esteem. In addition the participants' support and commitment to the group was demonstrated by high attendance to group sessions and their continued networking after the group sessions were over. Findings support the view that mild depression may lift over a period of six to eight weeks and that replication of the study should include moderately depressed women.

The third study, a replication of the intervention model, was conducted in the University of London with 20 moderately depressed middle-aged women. These volunteers were randomly selected and assigned to either the experimental or control condition. The treatment consisted of 14 weekly (two-hour) structured group sessions led by two professional nurses in London. Detailed description of methodology, findings as well as nurses' observation by the group's nurse-facilitators are included in the chapter. Again, statistically significant post-test differences between control and experimental groups were demonstrated for depression, self-esteem and hopelessness.

The following conclusions emerge:

1 Professional nurses (baccalaureate graduates) tend to be effective facilitators of depressed women's groups. Nurses' abilities to help women has been substantiated in these studies in the USA and the UK.
2 Coping strategies for women can be taught, tested and shared within a supportive group atmosphere.
3 Replication of the intervention model with increased numbers of women of a variety of ages and background could be useful future nursing research.

The significance of the intervention model is:

1 To help women cope effectively, take an active role in their own health.
2 To prevent possible severe depression in women.
3 To gain data about the complex phenomena of depression in women.
4 To strengthen the family unit by increased self-esteem of women.

Use of this approach by nurses already available in the community to provide women this assistance (by use of provided instruction manuals for the group facilitators as well as for each woman) could also reduce health care costs.

References

Back, K. W. and Taylor, R. (1976) Self-help groups: Tool or symbol? *Journal of Applied Behavioural Science*, 12: 295–309.

Bardwick, J. M. (1978) Middle age and a sense of future. *Merrill-Palmer Quarterly*, 24: 130–6.

Barrett, N. (1979) Women in the job market: Occupations, earnings and career opportunities, in R. Smith (ed.) *The Subtle Revolution: Women at Work*. Washington, D.C.: Urban Institute.

Bart, P. B. (1971) Depression in middle-aged women, in V. Gomich and B. Moran (eds) *Women in Sexist Society*. New York: Basic Books: 163–86.

Beck, A. T. (1972) Measuring depression: The depression inventory, in T. A. Williams, M. N. Katz and J. A. Shield (eds) *Recent Advances in the Psychobiology of the Depressive Illnesses*. Washington, D.C.: Government Printing Office.

Beck, A. T. (1978) *Depression: Causes and Treatment*. Philadelphia, PA: University of Pennsylvania Press.

Beck, A. T. and Beamesderfer, A. (1974) Assessment of depression, the depression inventories, in P. Pichot (ed.) *Psychological Measurements in Psychopharmacology and Modern Pharmacopsychiatry*, vol. 7. Basle: Karger.

Beck, A. T., Rush, A. J., Shaw, B. F. and Emery, G. (1979) *Cognitive Therapy of Depression*. New York: Guilford Press.

Belle, D. (1982) *Lives in Stress: Women and Depression*. Beverly Hills, CA: Sage Publications.

Bothwell, S. and Weissman, M. (1977) Social impairments four years after an acute depressive episode. *American Journal of Orthopsychiatry*, 47: 231–7.

Braillier, L. (1980) Holistic health practice: Expanding the role of the psychiatric–mental health nurse, in J. Lancaster (ed.) *Community Mental Health Nursing*. New York: Mosby.

Broverman, I. K., Broverman, D., Clarkson, F. E., Rosendrantz, P. and Vogel, S. R. (1970) Sex-role stereotypes and clinical judgments of mental health. *Journal of Counselling and Clinical Psychology*, 34: 1–7.

Brown, C. R. and Hellinger, M. L. (1975) Therapists' attitudes toward women. *Social Work*, 21: 266–70.

Brown, G. W., Bhrolchain, M. N. and Harris, T. (1975) Social class and psychiatric disturbance among women in an urban population. *Sociology*, 9: 225–54.

Carmen, E., Russo, N. F. and Miller, J. B. (1981) Inequality and women's mental health: An overview. *American Journal of Psychiatry*, 138: 1319–30.

Chenitz, W. C. (1979) Primary depression in older women: Are current theories and treatment of depression relevant to this age group? *Journal of Psychiatric Nursing and Mental Health Services*, 17–23.

Cherlin, A. J. (1981) *Marriage, Divorce, Remarriage.* Cambridge, MA: Harvard University Press.

Chodoff, P. (1972) The depressive personality. *Archives of General Psychiatry*, 27: 666–73.

Claerhout, S., Elder, J. and Carolyn, J. (1982) Problem-solving skills of rural battered women. *American Journal of Community Psychology*, 10(5): 605–606.

Clayton, P. J., Martin, S., Davis, M. and Wochnik, E. (1980) Mood disorders in women professionals. *Journal of Affective Disorders*, 2: 37–46.

Cohen, J. and Cohen, P. (1975) *Applied Multiple Regression/Correlation Analysis for the Behavioral Sciences.* New York: Wiley.

Cooperstock, R. (1979) A review of women's psychotropic drug use. *Canadian Journal of Psychiatry*, 24: 29–34.

Cronbach, L. J. and Furby, L. (1970) How should we measure 'change' – or should we? *Psychological Bulletin*, 74: 68–80.

Curlee, (1969) Alcoholism and the 'empty nest'. *Bulletin of Menninger Clinic*, 33: 165–70.

Davis, S. M. (1977) Women's liberation groups as a primary preventive mental health strategy. *Community Mental Health Journal*, 13: 219–28.

Derogatis, L. (1976) *SCL-90 (Revised Version) Manual-1.* Baltimore, MD: Johns Hopkins University School of Medicine.

Dinnauer, L., Miller, M. and Frankforter, M. (1981) Implementation strategies for an inpatient woman's support group. *Journal of Psychiatric Nursing and Mental Health Services*, 19: 13–16.

Dohrenwend, B. S. (1973) Social status and stressful life events. *Journal of Personality and Social Psychology*, 28: 225–35.

Editorial (1979) Hysterectomy and the quality of a woman's life. *Archives of International Medicine*, 139: 146.

Emery, G. (1981) *A New Beginning: How You Can Change Your Life Through Cognitive Therapy.* New York: Simon & Schuster.

Fiske, D. W., Hunt, H. F., Luborsky, L., Orne, T. M., Parloff, M. B., Reiser, M. F. and Tuma, A. H. (1970) Planning of research on effectiveness of psychotherapy. *Archives of General Psychiatry*, 22: 22.

Gallese, L. and Treuting, E. (1981) Help for rape victims through group therapy. *Journal of Psychiatric Nursing and Mental Health Services*, 19: 20–21.

Goldberg, A. (1973) Psychotherapy of narcissistic injuries. *Archives of General Psychiatry*, 28: 722–6.

Gordon, V. C. (1979) Women and divorce: Implications for nursing care, in O. O. Kjervik-Martinson (ed.) *Women in Stress: A Nursing Perspective.* New York: Appleton-Century-Croft: 259–76.

Gordon, V. C. (1982) Themes and cohesives observed in a depressed women's support group. *Issues in Mental Health Nursing*, 4: 115–25.

Gordon, V. and LeDray, L. (1985) Depression in women: The challenge of treatment and prevention. *Journal of Psychosocial Nursing and Mental Health Services*, 23: 26–34.

Gove, W. (1972) The relationship between sex roles, mental illness and marital status. *Social Forces*, 51: 34–44.

Guttentag, M., Slasin, S. and Belle, D. (1980) *The Mental Health of Women.* New York: Academic Press.

Hirschfield, R. M. (1980) In M. Scarf (ed.) *Unfinished Business: Pressure Points in the Lives of Women.* New York: Ballantine Books: 277.

Hollon, S. O. (1980) Beck's 'Significant Other' Form (unpublished).

Horney, K. (1967) *Feminine Psychology.* New York: W. W. Norton.

Johnson, K. K. (1979) Durkheim revisited: Why do women kill themselves? *Suicide and Life Threatening Behaviour*, 9: 145–53.

Kagan, J. and Moss, H. A. (1971) Birth to maturity, in J. M. Bardwick (ed.) *Psychology of Women*. New York: Harper & Row.

Kaslow, S. (1982) Marriage and intimacy: The surprising staying power of loveless marriages. *Ladies Home Journal*, 3: 41–48.

Kivett, V. R. (1979) Religious motivation in middle age: Correlates and implications. *Journal of Gerontology*, 34: 106–15.

Kjervik, D. K. and Palta, M. (1978) Sex-role stereotyping in assessments of mental health. *Nursing Research*, 27: 166–71.

LeDray, L. and Chaignot, M. (1980) Services of sexual assault victims in Hennepin County. *Evaluation and Change* (special issue) 131–4.

Lewinsohn, P., Sullivan, J. and Grosscup, S. (1982) Behavioral therapy: Clinical applications, in A. J. Rush (ed.) *Short Term Psychotherapies of Depression*. New York: The Guilford Press: 50–87.

Loomis, M. E. (1979) *Group Process for Nurses,* vol. 23. St. Louis, MO: Mosby.

Lopata, H. Z. (1971) Widows as a minority group. *The Gerontologist*, spring: 67–75.

Lowenthal, M. F. and Chiriboga, D. (1972) Transition to the empty nest: Crisis, challenge or relief? *Archives of General Psychiatry*, 26: 8–14.

McLachlan, J. F., Walderman, R. L., Birchmore, D. F. and Marsden, L. R. (1976) Self-evaluation, role satisfaction in the woman alcoholic. *The International Journal of Addictions*, 14(6): 809–32.

Martin, R. L., Roberts, W. V. and Clayton, P. J. (1980) Psychiatric status after hysterectomy. *Journal of the American Medical Association*, 244: 350–3.

Maykowsky, V. P. (1980) Stress and mental health of women: a discussion of research and issue, in M. Guttentag (ed.) *The Mental Health of Women*. New York: Academic Press.

Miller, J. (1976) *Toward a New Psychology of Women*. Boston, MA: Beacon Press.

Neuberry, P., Weissman, M. and Myers, J. (1979) Working wives and housewives: Do they differ in mental status and social adjustment? *American Journal of Orthopsychiatry*, 49: 282–90.

Neugarten, B., Wood, L., Krainer, R. and Loomis, B. (1963) Women's attitudes toward the menopause. *Vita Humana*, 6: 140–51.

Notman, M. (1979) Midlife concerns in women: Implications of the menopause. *American Journal of Psychiatry*, 136: 1270–4.

Notman, M., Nadelson, C. and Bennett, M. (1978) Achievement conflict in women. *Psychotherapy and Psychosomatics*, 29: 203–213.

Parloff, M. B. (1980) Psychotherapy and research: An anaclitic depression. *Psychiatry*, 43: 280.

Pilisuk, M. and Froland, C. (1978) Kinship, social network, social support and health. *Social Science and Medicine*, 12(B), 273–80.

Powell, B. (1977) The empty nest, employment, and psychiatric symptoms in college-educated women. *Psychology of Women Quarterly*, 2: 35–43.

Radloff, L. (1975) Sex differences in depression: The effects of occupation and marital status. *Sex Roles*, 1: 249–64.

Radloff, L. and Monroe, M. (1978) Sex differences in helplessness – with implications for depression, in L. Hansen and R. Rapoza (eds) *Career Development and Counseling of Women*. Springfield, IL: Thomas.

Radloff, L. S. and Rae, D. (1979) Susceptibility and precipitating factors in depression: Sex differences and similarities. *Journal of Abnormal Psychology*, 88: 174–81.

Raphael, B. (1976) Psychiatric aspects of hysterectomy, in J. G. Howell (ed.) *Modern Perspectives in the Psychiatric Aspects of Surgery*. New York: Brunner-Mazel.

Ryden, M. (1978) Coopersmith self-esteem inventory (adult version). *Psychological Reports*, 43: 1189–1190.

Sarason, I., Johnson, J. and Siegel, J. (1978) Assessing the impact of life changes: Development of the Life Experiences Survey. *Journal of Consulting and Clinical Psychology*, 46: 932–46.

Scarf, M. (1980) *Unfinished Business: Pressure Points in the Lives of Women.* New York: Ballantine Books.

Schaef, A. W. (1981) *Women's Reality.* Minneapolis, MN: Winston Press.

Schwab, J. J., Bralow, M. and Holzer, C. (1967) A comparison of two rating scales for depression. *Journal of Clinical Psychology*, 23: 94–96.

Seligman, M. E. (1975) *Helplessness.* San Francisco, CA: W. H. Freeman.

Shaw, B. F. (1977) Comparison of cognitive therapy and behavior therapy in the treatment of depression. *Journal of Consulting and Clinical Psychology*, 45: 543–51.

Shields, L. (1980) *Displaced Homemakers.* New York: McGraw-Hill.

Stevenson, J. (1977) *Issues and Crises During Middlescence.* New York: Appleton-Century-Crofts.

Thurnher, M. (1976) Midlife marriage: Sex differences in evaluation and perspectives. *International Journal of Aging and Human Development*, 7: 129–35.

Tubesing, D., Holinger, P., Westberg, G. and Lichter, E. (1977) The Wholistic Health Center Project. *Medical Care*, 15: 217-27.

Tucker, S. J. (1977) The menopause: How much soma and how much psyche? *JOGN Nursing*, 6: 40–47.

van Keep, P. and Prill, H. (1975) Psycho-sociology of menopause and post-menopause. *Frontiers in Hormone Research*, 3: 32–39.

van Servellen, G. and Dull, L. (1981) Group psychotherapy for depressed women: A model. *Journal of Psychiatric Nursing and Mental Health Services*, 19: 25–30.

Walker, L. E. (1979) *The Battered Woman.* New York: Harper & Row.

Weissman, M. M. and Paykel, E. S. (1974) *The Depressed Woman.* Chicago, IL: University of Chicago Press.

Weissman, M. M. and Klerman, G. L. (1977) Sex differences and the epidemiology of depression. *Archives of General Psychiatry*, 34: 98–111.

Weissman, M., Pincus, C., Radding, N., Lawrence, R. and Siegel, R. (1973) The educated housewife: Mild depression and the search for work. *American Journal of Orthopsychiatry*, 43(4): 565–73.

Wittenborn, J. R. and Buhler, R. (1979) Somatic discomforts among depressed women. *Archives of General Psychiatry*, 36: 465–71.

Wood, H. P. and Duffy, E. L. (1966) Psychological factors in alcoholic women. *American Journal of Psychiatry*, 123(3): 341–5.

Young, J. E. (1981) Cognitive therapy and loneliness, in G. Emery, S. Hollon, and R. Bedrosian (eds) *New Directions in Cognitive Therapy.* Guilford Press, New York.

THE MORTALITY OF DOCTORS IN RELATION TO THEIR SMOKING HABITS: A PRELIMINARY REPORT

Richard Doll and A. Bradford Hill

In the last five years a number of studies have been made of the smoking habits of patients with and without lung cancer (Doll and Hill 1950, 1952; Levin, Goldstein and Gerhardt 1950; Mills and Porter 1950; Schrek, Baker, Ballard and Dolgoff 1950; Wynder and Graham 1950; McConnell, Gordon and Jones 1952; Koulumies 1953; Sadowsky, Gilliam and Cornfield 1953; Wynder and Cornfield 1953; Breslow, Hoaglin, Rasmussen and Abrams 1954; Watson and Conte 1954). All these studies agree in showing that there are more heavy smokers and fewer non-smokers among patients with lung cancer than among patients with other diseases. With one exception (the difference between the proportions of non-smokers found by McConnell, Gordon and Jones 1952) these differences are large enough to be important. While, therefore, the various authors have all shown that there is an 'association' between lung cancer and the amount of tobacco smoked, they have differed in their interpretation. Some have considered that the only reasonable explanation is that smoking is a factor in the production of the disease; others have not been prepared to deduce causation and have left the association unexplained.

Further retrospective studies of that same kind would seem to us unlikely to advance our knowledge materially or to throw any new light upon the nature of the association. If, too, there were any undetected flaw in the evidence that such studies have produced, it would be exposed only by some entirely new approach. That approach we considered should be 'prospective'.[1] It should determine the frequency with which the disease appeared, in the future, among groups of persons whose smoking habits were already known.

Method of investigation

To derive such groups of persons with different smoking habits we wrote in October 1951 to the members of the medical profession in the United Kingdom and asked them to fill in a simple questionary. In addition to giving their name, address and age, the doctors were asked to classify themselves into one of three groups – namely, (1) whether they were, at that time, smoking; (2) whether they had smoked but had given up; or (3) whether they had never smoked regularly (that is, had never smoked as much as one cigarette a day, or its equivalent in pipe tobacco, for as long as one year). All present smokers and ex-smokers were asked additional questions. The former were asked the ages at which they had started smoking and the amount of tobacco that they were smoking, and the method by which it was consumed, at the time of replying to the questionary. The ex-smokers were asked similar questions but relating to the time at which they had last given up smoking.

The questionary was intentionally kept short and simple in the hope of encouraging a high proportion of replies, without which the inquiry must have failed. In a covering letter the doctors were invited to give any information on their smoking habits or history which might be of interest, but, apart from that, no information was asked for about previous changes in habit (other than the amount smoked prior to last giving up, if smoking had been abandoned). It was, of course, realized that the habits of early adult life might well be more relevant to the development of a disease with a long induction period than the most recent habits. On the other hand, we regarded the procedure adopted as justified, not only because of the extreme difficulty of obtaining sufficiently accurate records of past smoking habits, but also because of the experience of our previous retrospective investigation (Doll and Hill 1952). This investigation, in which nearly 5,000 patients were interviewed, had shown that the classification of smokers according to the amount that they had most recently smoked gave almost as sharp a differentiation between the groups of patients with and without lung cancer as the use of smoking histories over many years – theoretically more relevant statistics, but clearly based on less accurate data.

From their replies to the questionary the doctors were classified into broad groups according to age, the amount of tobacco smoked, the method of smoking, and whether smoking had been continued or abandoned. These groups, based upon smoking habits at the end of 1951, form the 'exposed to risk'.

To complete the investigation it was necessary to obtain information about the causes of death of all those doctors who had replied to the questionary and who subsequently died. Through the courtesy of the Registrars-General in the United Kingdom[2] a form showing particulars of the cause of death has been provided for every death of a doctor registered since the questionary was sent out. Each form relating to a doctor who had completed the questionary has been extracted and allocated to the smoking group in which that doctor had previously been placed. Hence it has been possible to calculate the death rates from different causes within each of the main smoking categories.

The exposed to risk

The questionary was sent out on 31 October, 1951 to 59,600 men and women on the *Medical Register*. Of the 41,024 replies received, 40,564 were sufficiently complete to be utilized. Of this total, however, 10,017

Table 9.1 Amount of tobacco smoked: Male doctors aged 35 years and above

| Age in years | No. of non-smokers | No. of men smoking* a daily average of: | | | Total no. of men |
		1 g.–†	15 g.–	25 g.+	
35–44	1,457 (16.3%)	2,864 (32.1%)	2,888 (32.4%)	1,716 (19.2%)	8,925 (100.0%)
45–54	835 (11.7%)	2,087 (29.2%)	2,332 (32.7%)	1,886 (26.4%)	7,140 (100.0%)
55–64	377 (9.3%)	1,376 (33.9%)	1,283 (31.6%)	1,027 (25.3%)	4,063 (100.1%)
65–74	231 (8.6%)	1,218 (45.2%)	807 (30.0%)	438 (16.3%)	2,694 (100.1%)
75–84	164 (11.8%)	768 (55.3%)	326 (23.5%)	132 (9.5%)	1,390 (100.1%)
85 and above	29 (16.4%)	118 (66.7%)	26 (14.7%)	4 (2.3%)	177 (100.1%)
All ages (Crude %)	3,093 (12.7%)	8,431 (34.6%)	7,662 (31.4%)	5,203 (21.3%)	24,389 (100.0%)

Notes: * The figures include (1) men smoking the given amounts at the end of 1951, and (2) ex-smokers smoking the given amounts at the time they gave up smoking.
† 1 cigarette equals 1 g.; 1 oz. of tobacco a week taken to equal 4 g. a day.

Table 9.2 Method of smoking: Male doctors aged 35 years and above

| Age in years | No. of men smoking | | | Total no. of smokers |
	Pipes	Pipes and cigarettes*	Cigarettes	
35–44	1,001 (13.4%)	1,240 (16.6%)	5,227 (70.0%)	7,468 (100.0%)
45–54	843 (13.4%)	1,301 (20.6%)	4,161 (66.0%)	6,305 (100.0%)
55–64	630 (17.1%)	991 (26.9%)	2,065 (56.0%)	3,686 (100.0%)
65–74	601 (24.4%)	661 (26.8%)	1,201 (48.8%)	2,463 (100.0%)
75–84	411 (33.5%)	288 (23.5%)	527 (43.0%)	1,226 (100.0%)
85 and above	72 (48.6%)	23 (15.5%)	53 (35.8%)	148 (99.9%)
All ages (Crude %)	3,558 (16.7%)	4,504 (21.2%)	13,234 (62.1%)	21,296 (100.0%)

Note: * The few men who smoked cigars have been classed as mixed pipe and cigarette smokers.

related to men under the age of 35 and 6,158 to women of all ages. Since lung cancer is relatively uncommon in women and rare in men under 35, useful figures are unlikely to be obtained in these groups for some years to come. In this preliminary report we have therefore confined our attention to men aged 35 and above. The numbers of them who had (1) never smoked regularly, (2) smoked greater or less amounts of tobacco, or (3) smoked cigarettes or pipes or both cigarettes and pipes are shown in Tables 9.1 and 9.2. It will be seen that in this population the distribution of smoking habits varies considerably with age. Since cancer incidence also varies greatly with age it will be necessary to use death rates at specific ages, or a rate standardized for age, when comparing the mortality among the men in the different smoking categories.

It may well be that the smoking habits of the 40,564 doctors who replied to us are not representative of the smoking habits of all doctors. One category may have tended to reply more readily than another. We shall not, however, need to use the replies in total but always separately within the four smoking divisions. All that we require are sufficient numbers within each of those divisions.

Table 9.3 Criteria on which diagnosis of primary lung cancer was established

Diagnostic criteria	No. of cases	% of total
1 Histological evidence of carcinoma, plus evidence of the site of the primary tumour from necropsy, operation, bronchoscopy, or radiological examination	21*	58
2 Evidence of the site of the primary tumour from operation (2), bronchoscopy (3), or radiological examination (7), without histological evidence	12	33
3 Evidence from clinical examination only	3	9
All cases	36	100

* 7 squamous-cell carcinoma, 9 oat-cell and anaplastic carcinoma, 3 adenocarcinoma, and 2 cell type undetermined.

The deaths

In the 29 months that have elapsed since the questionaries were sent out (November 1951 to March 1954 inclusive), 789 deaths have been reported among the male doctors who were aged 35 years and above at the time that they completed the questionary. Of these deaths, 35 were certified as due to lung cancer; in one further case lung cancer was reported as contributing to death without being the direct cause. We wrote to the doctor certifying the cause of death in each of these 36 cases and asked him to tell us the nature of the evidence upon which his diagnosis was based. The information received is analysed in Table 9.3. There were firm grounds for the diagnosis in at least 33 of the cases, and in only three was the evidence limited to clinical examination.

Preliminary results

Amount of smoking

Death rates from six groups of diseases have been calculated for each of the categories of men classified as non-smokers or as having smoked greater or smaller amounts of tobacco. The rates have been standardized for age (by the direct method), using the total male population of the United Kingdom on 31 December, 1951 as the standard population.[3] The resulting annual rates for each smoking category from all causes of death and from six causes separately are shown in Table 9.4. It will be seen that the death rate from lung cancer increased steadily from 0.00 per 1,000 in non-smokers to 1.14 per 1,000 among the men recorded as having smoked 25 or more grams of tobacco daily. A similar but less steep rise is also seen in the death rate from coronary thrombosis (from 3.89 per 1,000 in non-smokers to 5.15 in the heaviest smokers). In the other disease groups the changes in mortality are irregular and, for the most part, small.

The statistical significance of these differences in the death rates can be

Table 9.4 Standardized death rate per annum per 1,000 men aged 35 years and above in relation to the most recent amount of tobacco smoked

Cause of death	No of deaths recorded	Death rates of non-smokers	Death rates of men smoking a daily average of			Death rate of all men
			1 g.–	15 g.–	25 g.+	
Lung cancer	36*	0.00	0.48	0.67	1.14	0.66
Other cancers	92	2.32	1.41	1.50	1.91	1.65
Respiratory disease (other than cancer)	54	0.86	0.88	1.01	0.77	0.94
Coronary thrombosis	235	3.89	3.91	4.71	5.15	4.27
Other cardiovascular diseases	126*	2.23	2.07	1.58	2.78	2.14
Other diseases	247	4.27	4.67	3.91	4.52	4.36
All causes	789	13.61	13.42	13.38	16.30	14.00

* 1 case in which lung cancer was recorded as a contributory but not a direct cause of death has been entered in both groups.

more easily assessed from the actual numbers of deaths recorded; that is, by comparing them with the numbers which would have been expected to occur in each smoking category if smoking were quite unrelated to the chance of dying of lung cancer. For example, 13 men aged 55–64 when the questionary was completed subsequently died of lung cancer. The proportions of all the men in this age group who were non-smokers, smoked 1–14 grams a day, 15–24 grams a day, or 25 or more grams a day were 9.3 per cent, 33.9 per cent, 31.6 per cent, and 25.3 per cent. If the mortality from lung cancer is unrelated to smoking, then the 13 deaths should be distributed to the smoking groups in these ratios. Similar calculations have been made for the numbers of men dying of lung cancer in the other age groups – namely, one at ages 35–44, eight at ages 45–54, six at ages 65–74, and eight at ages 75–84. The total numbers of deaths expected in each smoking category were then obtained by adding the numbers for the separate age groups. The results were as follows:

	Non-smokers	Smokers of a daily average of			Total
		1 g.–	15 g.–	25 g.+	
Observed deaths	0	12	11	13	36
Expected deaths	3.77	14.20	10.73	7.33	36.03

These differences between the observed and expected deaths are statistically significant ($\chi^2 = 8.5$, $n = 3$, $P = 0.04$). We may note, too, that the ordinary χ^2 test of significance fails to take into account the biologically important finding that there is a continuous increase in the proportion of observed to expected deaths as the amount of tobacco smoked increases – a finding which makes it possible to attach a simple interpretation to the results.[4]

In none of the other disease groups are the differences between the observed and expected number of deaths found to be significant. The continuous change in the ratio between the observed and expected deaths from coronary thrombosis is, however, suggestive.[5] For all causes of death taken together, there is an excess mortality among smokers of 25 or more grams a day and a corresponding deficiency of deaths, almost equally divided, among the non-smokers and the men in the less heavy smoking categories. The differences are statistically significant ($\chi^2 = 8.8$, $n = 3$, $P = 0.03$). When, however, the lung cancer deaths are omitted, the differences are no longer significant ($\chi^2 = 6.5$, $n = 3$, $P = 0.09$).

The distinction between the systematic variation in the mortality from lung cancer with the amount smoked and the irregular (or small) variation observed in the other disease groups studied is perhaps shown more clearly in Figure 9.1.

Method of smoking

With the very simple form of questionary that we deliberately employed we can distinguish the different types of smokers only according to whether they were smokers of cigarettes, of pipes, or of both cigarettes and pipes, at a given point of time – that is, for smokers at the time they filled in the questionary and for ex-smokers at the time that they had previously given up smoking. It is clear, therefore, that the real numbers of 'pure' cigarette smokers and of 'pure' pipe smokers must be less, and, almost certainly, appreciably less, than those we have allocated to those groups. Evidence of this was, in fact, provided by some doctors who volunteered additional information that they had in previous years smoked their tobacco by different methods and in different amounts. Any real difference between the risks associated with cigarette and with pipe smoking must therefore be blurred in our figures, since each group will contain men who have also been exposed, in part, to whatever risks may be associated with the other type of smoking.

With that very material proviso in mind, we note that, of the 36 men with lung cancer, 25 had reported themselves as cigarette smokers, four as pipe smokers, and seven as smokers of both cigarettes and pipes. If the method of smoking were entirely unassociated with the risks of lung cancer we would have expected (by the method of calculation described above) these 36 cases to be subdivided in the following proportions: 19.6 cigarette smokers, 7.6 pipe smokers, 8.8 cigarette and pipe smokers. While there is an observed excess of cigarette smokers and a deficit of pipe smokers amongst the deaths, the differences are not statistically significant ($\chi^2 = 3.5$, $n = 2$, $P > 0.10$), and with the present number of deaths it has not been possible to allow adequately for differences in the amount smoked.

In none of the other five disease groups studied was there a significant difference between the observed and expected deaths for the different types of smokers, and the actual differences were, in fact, smaller than those we have reported above for the deaths from lung cancer.

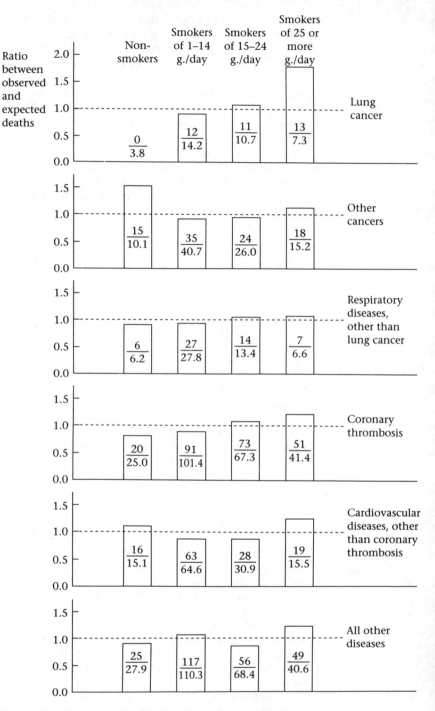

Figure 9.1 Variation in mortality with amount smoked

Note: The ordinate shows the ratio between the number of deaths observed and the number expected (as entered in each column).

Comparison between the results of the retrospective and prospective inquiries

The relative excess of cigarette smokers and the corresponding deficit of pipe smokers in the 36 cancer of the lung deaths amongst the doctors, though not formally significant, at least does not run counter to the tentative conclusion of a lower risk to pipe smokers that we drew from the data obtained from hospital patients. More striking, however, is the similarity we find in the two inquiries in the upward trend of the death rate from cancer of the lung that accompanies increased *amount* of smoking. In our previous 'backward' inquiry we made estimates of the death rates among residents in Greater London in 1950 who had smoked different quantities of tobacco. These estimates we have now recalculated to bring them into line with the slightly different methodology of our present analysis – that is, we have limited the rates to ages 45–74, we have standardized them on the total male population of the UK at 31 December, 1951 and we have based them upon the most recent smoking history of the patient instead of upon a longer-term history. The results, together with the corresponding figures for doctors, are set out in Table 9.5.

The actual rates for the doctors are, it will be seen, very materially less than those we have estimated for the males of Greater London. On the other hand, there is a remarkable similarity in the increases in mortality from non-smokers to 'light' smokers, from 'light' smokers to 'medium' smokers, and finally, from 'medium' smokers to 'heavy' smokers. In the 'backward' group the percentages of the average rate are 6, 79, 112 and 203; in the 'forward' group they are 0, 68, 133 and 199. Remembering that at these ages we have only 27 deaths of doctors to analyse, the similarity is perhaps too good to be true; it may well be due partly to

Table 9.5 Standardized death rates from cancer of the lung per 1000 men aged 45–74 years in relation to the most recent amount of tobacco smoked, estimated from (1) the 'backward' inquiry into the histories of patients with cancer of the lung and other diseases in London (1952), and (2) from the present 'forward' inquiry into the mortality of doctors (1954)

		Smokers of:			
	Non-smokers	1–14 g./day	15–24 g./day	25 g. +/day	All groups*
Standardized rates					
'Backward' study of patients' histories	0.11	1.56	2.20	4.00	1.97
'Forward' study of mortality of doctors	0.00	0.50	0.97	1.45	0.73
Each rate as % of the rate for all groups					
'Backward' study of patients' histories	6%	79%	112%	203%	100%
'Forward' study of mortality of doctors	0%	68%	133%	199%	100%

Note: * The unweighted average of the four rates.

chance. We would, however, suggest that it is at least reasonable to conclude that there is no incompatibility between the results of the two
inquiries in their measurements of the increase of mortality from lung
cancer in relation to the increases in smoking.

The incompatibility lies, as observed above, in the actual level of the
rates in the two inquiries. Why should the rates for the doctors be so
much lower? One important reason – and one which applies to all causes
of death and not only to lung cancer – is, we believe, that doctors who
were already ill of a disease likely to prove fatal within a short space
of time would have been disinclined, or indeed unable, to answer our
inquiries. In other words, we should learn of their deaths, but we would
have no corresponding completed questionary on our files. That this may
well be true is shown (1) by the relatively low death rate from all causes
that we have recorded – namely, 14.0 per 1,000 per annum, against 24.6
per 1,000 for men of all social classes in the same age group in the UK
in 1951, and (2) by the fact that over the 29 months of the investigation
there has been a rise in the proportion of the deaths sent to us by the
Registrars-General for which we have been able to find a completed
questionary. If persons sick of a fatal illness were unwilling to reply, or,
indeed, never saw our communication, that bias would tend to wear off
with the passage of time – as it shows signs of doing.

The question is whether such a bias would differentially affect the
mortality of the smoking group. Could it artificially produce the gradient
that we have observed with cancer of the lung, and probably with coronary thrombosis, whilst not producing any gradient with other causes of
death? For such an effect we should have to suppose that the heavier
smokers who already knew that they had cancer of the lung tended to
reply more often than non-smokers, or lighter smokers, in a similar situation. That would not seem probable to us. As evidence to the contrary
we would also add (1) that, although the numbers of deaths are admit-
tedly very small, we have not seen any obvious change in the lung cancer
gradient over the 29 months of the inquiry, and (2) that it would be
surprising if a gradient produced in this way so closely resembled the
gradient we obtained in our retrospective inquiry.

Other factors than this may have contributed to the lower death rates
from cancer of the lung recorded for the doctors. There may well be
differences between them and our male London patients in methods of
smoking (use of pipes as against cigarettes), and there may be differences
in the age of starting to smoke. The London rates are, too, we know,
higher than the rates for the country as a whole, and it was from the
latter that the doctors were drawn.

The diagnoses

It might perhaps be argued that physicians in reaching a diagnosis of
cancer of the lung have been biased by the patient's smoking history. We
have, however, already shown in Table 9.3 that there was little doubt of
the diagnosis in the great majority of the deaths. That would not, of

course, meet the point that the physician might take more active steps to make a diagnosis in a heavy smoker than in a light or non-smoker, but, if that were the case, deaths from other causes would have to be proportionately less in the groups of heavier smokers. There is certainly no sign of that in our present figures, and the steadiness of the upward gradient among smokers would seem to make such a bias very unlikely.

Conclusion

If, as we think, the association between smoking and the disease is real and not due to some such bias as we have discussed, it is likely that the increase in mortality with the amount smoked is, in fact, greater than that indicated by our present figures. The rates we give were calculated from the limited data obtained in reply to a simple questionary, and related (apart from non-smokers) to smoking habits at a single point of time. No attention was paid to the changes in smoking history that many men experience – even when we had evidence of such changes. Consequently the group of doctors classified by us as light smokers (smokers of 1–14 grams a day) may well contain an appreciable proportion of persons who have for many years – and possibly for the more relevant years – smoked larger amounts of tobacco; and (perhaps to a less extent) the group of heavy smokers (smokers of 25 or more grams a day) may contain men who for the most part of their lives have smoked much less.

Evidence of these changes was provided, as pointed out previously in relation to the relative risks of cigarette and pipe smoking, by some doctors who volunteered statements on their forms that they had previously smoked different amounts of tobacco. We know, for instance, that among those who subsequently developed lung cancer one had been smoking 25 cigarettes a day and 1 ounce of pipe tobacco a week until he cut down to 12 cigarettes a day on his retirement in 1945. Another had changed from 25 to 30 cigarettes a day to five ounces of pipe tobacco a week (equivalent to 20 cigarettes a day) in September 1951. In another instance, the doctor had described himself as smoking 3.5 ounces of pipe tobacco a week, but a friend, who signed the death certificate and had known him for 25 years, stated he had previously been one of the heaviest smokers of both cigarettes and pipe he had ever known. Such factors not only could not produce an exaggeration of the true relationship but must lead to an understatement of it by inflating the mortality among light smokers and reducing the mortality among heavy smokers.

The investigation has not, as yet, continued long enough to show whether there is a relationship between smoking and the mortality from any other disease, but from the preliminary figures it would seem unlikely that there is any as close as that observed with lung cancer. The numbers of deaths, however, from some potentially interesting diseases are as yet small (for example, from cancer of the buccal cavity and larynx and from duodenal ulcer). There have, on the other hand, been a large number of deaths attributable to coronary thrombosis. It seems clear that smoking cannot be a major factor in their production, but the steady increase in mortality with the amount of tobacco smoking recorded suggests that there is a subgroup of these cases in which tobacco has a significant adjuvant effect.

Summary

At the end of 1951 some 40,000 men and women on the British *Medical Register* replied to a simple questionary relating to their smoking habits. On that basis they were divided into non-smokers and three groups of smokers (including ex-smokers) according to the amount they smoked at that time (or when they gave up).

The certified causes of death of those men and women who have since died have been supplied by the Registrars-General of the UK over the ensuing 29 months. This preliminary report is confined to the deaths among the 24,389 men over the age of 35.

Though the numbers of deaths at present available are small the resulting rates reveal a significant and steadily rising mortality from deaths due to cancer of the lung as the amount of tobacco smoked increases. There is also a rise in the mortality from deaths attributed to coronary thrombosis as the amount smoked increases, but the gradient is much less steep than that revealed by cancer of the lung. The other groups of deaths so far analysed reveal no gradient (other forms of cancer, other forms of cardiovascular disease, respiratory diseases, all other causes).

The figures for cancer of the lung are in conformity with those found previously in an extensive inquiry into the smoking histories of patients with cancer of the lung and with other diseases.

The death rates of doctors reported here are, almost certainly, artificially low. There is evidence that this is due to a reluctance, or inability, of persons suffering from a fatal illness to reply to the questionary. In spite of this defect and the present small numbers of deaths, we thought it necessary, in view of the nature of the results, to lay these preliminary observations before the survivors of the 40,000 men and women who made them possible.

Acknowledgement

We are most grateful to the British Medical Association for having dispatched the questionaries and letters to the doctors on our behalf; to the individual doctors for having completed the questionaries; and to those practitioners and consultants to whom we wrote for details of the evidence on which the diagnosis of lung cancer was made. We are deeply indebted to the Registrars-General of the United Kingdom for information about the deaths of doctors. We also offer our thanks to Dr P. Armitage, who suggested the use of Yates's method of assessing the significance of a trend, and to Mrs Joan Bodington, Miss Muriel Greening and Miss Keena Jones for the onerous work of filing, coding, and enumerating the questionaries.

Notes

1 *O.E.D.* Characterized by looking forward into the future. (Leigh Hunt: 'He was a retrospective rather than a prospective man.')
2 The Registrars-General of England and Wales, Scotland, Northern Ireland, the Isle of Man, Jersey and Guernsey.
3 Thus for each of the four smoking categories in Table 9.1 death rates were separately calculated, for each age group. These age rates were then applied to the corresponding UK populations in 1951 to reach the death rate at all ages that would have prevailed in the UK population if it had experienced the various rates at ages of a particular smoking group.
4 The present data provide a special case of the general problem of assessing the significance of a trend, considered by Yates (1948). By his method we obtain $\chi^2 = 7.7$, $n = 1$, $P < 0.01$.
5 By Yates's method it is statistically significant; $\chi^2 = 4.6$, $n = 1$, $P = 0.03$.

References

Breslow, L., Hoaglin, Le M., Rasmussen, G. and Abrams, H. K. (1954) *American Journal of Public Health*, 44, 171.
Doll, R. and Hill, A. B. (1950) *British Medical Journal*, 2, 739.
Doll, R. and Hill, A. B. (1952) *British Medical Journal*, 2, 1271.
Koulumies, M. (1953) *Acta Radiol., Stockh.*, 39, 255.
Levin, M. L., Goldstein, H. and Gerhardt, P. R. (1950) *Journal of the American Medical Association*, 143, 336.
McConnell, R. B., Gordon, K. C. T. and Jones, T. (1952) *Lancet*, 2, 651.
Mills, C. A. and Porter, M. M. (1950) *Cancer Res.*, 10, 539.
Sadowsky, D. A., Gilliam, A. G. and Cornfield, J. (1953) *Journal of the National Cancer Institute*, 13, 1237.
Schrek, R., Baker, L. A., Ballard, G. P. and Dolgoff, S. (1950) *Cancer Res.*, 10, 49.
Watson, W. L. and Conte, A. J. (1954) *Cancer*, 7, 245.
Wynder, E. L. and Cornfield, J. (1953) *New England Journal of Medicine*, 248, 441.
Wynder, E. L. and Graham, E. A. (1950) *Journal of the American Medical Association*, 143, 329.
Yates, F. (1948) *Biometrika*, 35, 176.

ETHNIC VARIATION IN THE FEMALE LABOUR FORCE: A RESEARCH NOTE

Pamela Abbott and Melissa Tyler

Abstract

The 1991 Census question on ethnic origin makes it possible to analyse occupational segregation by gender and ethnic group in a way which has not been feasible before. The analysis shows that Black Caribbean and African women are more likely to be economically active that White ones (i.e. employed or seeking employment). It confirms that all non-White women are more likely than White ones to be unemployed or on a government scheme. However, it reveals considerable variation between ethnic groups and does not confirm any tendency for non-White women to be segregated uniformly in the 'lower' employment grades. Indeed, Pakistani and Chinese women are notably overrepresented in the managerial and professional grades, and more Chinese women than Chinese men are employed professionals or managers or owners of small businesses.

Introduction

Until recently it has been difficult, if not impossible, to look at the occupational characteristics of ethnic groups in any detail. The national surveys carried out regularly by PEP (Political and Economic Planning, later PSI, Policy Studies Institute), though covering large samples, were not sufficiently large to permit detailed analysis by occupational or ethnic group even for men and provided little information at all on working women (see Smith and McIntosh 1974; Smith 1976, 1977; Brown 1984). The Labour Force Survey has had a question on ethnic origin for some time, but again the sample size is too small to permit anything more than

Table 10.1 Employment status of men and women aged 16+

Status	Total (%)	Men (%)	Women (%)
Economically active	61	73	50
Of whom:			
In employment	55	65	46
Of those in employment:			
FT employed (31+ hours)	76	93	57
PT employed (30 or less)	22	4	41
Hours not classified	2	3	2
As proportion of category:			
FT employed (31+ hours) %		65	35
PT employed (30 or less) %		11	89
Total employees %		52.9	47.1

Note: In this and most subsequent tables, percentages are rounded to the nearest whole number. An asterisk indicates a percentage smaller than 0.5%
FT = full-time; PT = part-time
Source: derived from OPCS (1993a) Table 72

very broad classification of ethnic groups and their occupations, even using three-year aggregate data (DOE 1991: 65, 1993: 39; Sly 1994: 153). In 1991, however, the UK Population Census included a question on ethnic origin for the first time, permitting the examination in some detail of occupational distribution by gender and ethnic group.

Even with census data, it must be acknowledged that ethnic minorities constitute *very* small groups within the workforce. Thus in the 1991 Census 96 per cent of women in employment were classified as White, 1.5 per cent as Black, 1.8 per cent as Asian, 0.2 per cent as Chinese and 0.3 per cent as 'other'. The Census provides an opportunity not only to examine any changes in gendered segregation in the labour market since 1981 but also to look at ethnic variation in women's employment patterns – separately for ethnic groups, rather than aggregating people of very disparate backgrounds into the single category of 'Black'.

It is well established that women's patterns of labour market participation differ from men's. Women work in a narrower range of occupations than men, and this is especially true of part-time women employees. Just over 40 per cent of women employees work part-time, compared with not much more than 4 per cent of men, and women make up nine-tenths of all employed part-time workers (OPCS 1993a; see Table 10.1).

Women's employment status varies by ethnic group, however. Black Caribbean and non-Muslim Asian women are more likely to be economically active – employed or seeking work – than White women and, if employed, are more likely to be in full-time employment (see Table 10.2). Black women are also less likely to be working part-time than White women. About 40 per cent of White women employees are in part-time work, compared with about 21 per cent of Black Caribbean and Black African women, 24 per cent of Indian women, 27 per cent of Pakistani

Table 10.2 Economic activity as a percentage of the total population of women aged 16+, by ethnic group

Ethnic group	Percentage of total female population who are economically active	Percentage of eligible[1] female population who are economically active
All	50	73
White	50	69
Black (Caribbean)	67	82
Black (African)	60	74
Black (other)	63	76
Indian	55	82
Pakistani	27	32
Bangladeshi	22	28
Chinese	53	68
Other Asian	54	64
Other	50	68

Note: [1] That is, excluding inactive students, the permanently sick or disabled and retired women
Source: derived from OPCS (1993b) Table 10

Table 10.3 Full and part-time women employees as a percentage of women aged 16+ in employment, by ethnic group

Ethnic group	Full-time	Part-time
All (%)	61	39
White (%)	60	40
Black (Caribbean) (%)	79	21
Black (African) (%)	78	22
Black (other) (%)	78	22
Indian (%)	76	24
Pakistani (%)	73	27
Bangladeshi (%)	73	27
Chinese (%)	66	34
Other Asian (%)	75	25
Other (%)	73	27

Source: derived from OPCS (1993b) Table 10

and Bangladeshi women and nearly 34 per cent of Chinese women (Table 10.3).

All non-White women are more likely than White ones to be unemployed or on a government scheme. Seven per cent of economically active women aged 16 or over were classified as unemployed in the Census, and just over 1 per cent were on a government scheme. However, all non-White women, with the exception of Chinese women, were at least twice as likely to be unemployed as White women, and the same

Table 10.4 Women aged 16+ on government schemes or unemployed as a percentage of those economically active, by ethnic group

Ethnic group	On government schemes	Unemployed
All (%)	1.2	6.8
White (%)	1.1	6.3
Black (Caribbean) (%)	2.3	13.5
Black (African) (%)	4.3	24.7
Black (other) (%)	3.7	18.3
Indian (%)	2.0	12.7
Pakistani (%)	4.9	29.6
Bangladeshi (%)	7.9	34.5
Chinese (%)	1.8	8.3
Other Asian (%)	2.9	12.6
Other (%)	2.7	14.8

Source: derived from OPCS (1993b) Table 10

Table 10.5 Self-employed women as a percentage of those in employment, by ethnic group

Ethnic group	Total self-employed	With employees	Without employees
All (%)	6.7	2.3	4.3
White (%)	6.6	2.4	4.1
Black (Caribbean) (%)	2.0	0.6	1.4
Black (African) (%)	4.0	1.2	2.8
Black (other) (%)	4.1	1.1	3.0
Indian (%)	12.7	5.0	7.7
Pakistani (%)	15.6	5.7	9.9
Bangladeshi (%)	8.8	4.3	4.5
Chinese (%)	20.3	10.4	9.9
Other Asian (%)	6.9	2.8	4.4
Other (%)	7.2	2.0	5.2

Source: derived from OPCS (1993b) Table 10

was true of their likelihood of being on a government training scheme (Table 10.4).

About 7 per cent of all women in employment are self-employed – about a third with employees. Indian, Pakistani and Asian women are overrepresented in this category both as employers and as self-employed people without employees. Black Caribbean, Black African and other Black women are underrepresented in these 'self-employed' categories (Table 10.5).

It is evident from the Census data that, while there has been some reduction in horizontal and vertical gender segregation by occupation,

Table 10.6 Changes in gender segregation in the labour market, 1981–91

Socioeconomic group	Males			Females		
	1981 (%)	1991 (%)	% change	1981 (%)	1991 (%)	% change
Employers and managers:						
Large establishments	6	6	120	2	3	152
Small establishments	9	13	137	5	7	162
Professional workers:						
Self-employed	1	1	150	*	*	300
Employees	5	6	121	1	2	200
Other non-manual:						
Intermediate	8	10	132	15	18	123
Junior	10	9	93	39	37	94
Personal service	1	1	116	12	8	68
Manual workers:						
Foremen and supervisors	4	3	84	1	1	114
Skilled	27	20	77	4	3	66
Semi-skilled	14	12	82	11	9	86
Unskilled	6	4	68	7	7	106
Own account	6	9	160	2	3	145
Farming:						
Managers	1	1	86	*	*	100
Own account	1	1	100	*	*	200
Labourers	1	1	75	1	1	71
Armed forces	2	1	88	*	*	50

Note: The % change columns show the 1991 figure as a percentage of the 1981 figure, so that a figure of 100 indicates no change in either direction. (Because the percentages in the rest of the table have been rounded to whole numbers, the % change figure will seldom be precisely calculable from them.)
Source: derived from OPCS (1984) Table 17 and OPCS (1993a) Table 92

continuing a trend noted throughout this century (Hakim 1979; Abbott and Sapsford 1987), the reduction is slow and the degree of segregation still very marked (see Table 10.6). In 1991 women made up 76 per cent of all junior non-manual workers and 82 per cent of all personal service workers, whereas men constituted over 80 per cent of professional workers, foremen and supervisors, skilled manual workers, 'own account' manual workers, farmers and members of the armed forces. Only in routine non-manual and unskilled manual work did the proportion of women in the category exceed their proportion overall in the workforce (44 per cent). Furthermore, 63 per cent of employed women are in routine non-manual work (see Table 10.7). The 1991 Census enables us to see if there are variations in horizontal and vertical occupational segregation between women from different ethnic groups.

The tables in Appendix A give details of women's ethnic group by

Table 10.7 Labour market distribution by gender in the UK, 1991

Socioeconomic group	Men (%)	Women (%)	Percentages of total group:	
			Men	Women
Employers and managers:				
Large establishments	6	3	71	29
Small establishments	12	7	69	31
Professional workers:				
Self-employed	2	*	87	13
Employees	6	2	82	18
Other non-manual:				
Intermediate	10	18	41	59
Junior	9	36	24	76
Personal services	1	8	18	82
Manual workers:				
Foremen and supervisors	3	1	84	16
Skilled	20	3	91	9
Semi-skilled	11	9	61	39
Unskilled	4	7	41	59
Own account	9	3	80	20
Farming:				
Employers and managers	1	*	86	14
Own account	1	*	86	14
Labourers	1	1	70	30
Armed forces	1	*	92	8

Note: Of those classified as 'in employment' in the original table, 1.0 per cent of men and 0.8 per cent of women were 'unclassifiable', and 1.6 per cent of men and 1.2 per cent of women were on government schemes. These are not shown in the table above but have been included in the total on which the percentages are based
Source: derived from OPCS (1993a) Table 92

occupational group. Asian and Chinese women are underrepresented as employers and managers of large establishments but overrepresented as employers in small establishments and as self-employed or employee professional workers. Black Caribbean and Black African women are over-represented in intermediate non-manual work, whereas Indian, Pakistani, Bangladeshi and Chinese women are underrepresented. Chinese women are especially underrepresented in the 'junior non-manual' category, but all other groups with the exception of 'White' and 'Black other' are somewhat overrepresented. Bangladeshi, Chinese, 'other Asian' and Black African women are overrepresented in personal service work, and Indian and Pakistani women underrepresented. Indian, Pakistani and Bangladeshi women are overrepresented in the skilled and semi-skilled manual cat-egories, and Black Caribbean women are also overrepresented in the semi-skilled category and Black African women in the unskilled category. Chinese women are notably underrepresented in all manual categories

Table 10.8 Women in routine non-manual work, by ethnic group

Ethnic group	Percentage of ethnic group in routine non-manual work
All	63
White	64
Black (Caribbean)	67
Black (African)	63
Black (other)	67
Indian	48
Pakistani	50
Bangladeshi	61
Chinese	57
Other Asian	66
Other	67

Source: derived from OPCS (1993b) Table 16

except 'own account' manual work, where they are grossly overrepresented (along with Pakistani women).

So patterns of occupational segregation do vary for women by ethnic group, but within the overall pattern of the gendered and segregated labour market. For example, 63 per cent of all employed women are in routine non-manual work, compared with 20 per cent of employed men. When this is disaggregated by ethnic group (Table 10.8), it is evident that this concentration of women in routine non-manual work is common across ethnic groups. There is, however, some variation; for example, only 48 per cent of women of Indian origin are in routine non-manual work, compared with 67 per cent of Black Caribbean women.

Similarly, women are more likely to be in semi- or unskilled than in skilled manual work, regardless of ethnicity. However, Indian, Bangladeshi and Pakistani women are overrepresented in skilled and semi-skilled manual work and underrepresented in the unskilled category, while Chinese women are underrepresented in all categories of manual work except 'own account' work (see Table 10.9).

Overall, women are underrepresented in professional and managerial work, less than 13 per cent of employed women being found there. Black Caribbean women are notably underrepresented, however, and Pakistani and Chinese women are notably overrepresented. When we examine this band of occupations in more detail (Table 10.10) we can see some interesting variation, but it is only Chinese women who are overrepresented compared with men in any professional or managerial work – 15 per cent of Chinese women are employers or managers in small establishments, compared with 13 per cent of men, and over 7 per cent are employed professionals, compared with less than 6 per cent of employed men.

To summarize: 69 per cent of eligible White women aged 16 or over are in the labour force, of whom approximately 40 per cent work part-time, 7 per cent are recorded by the Census as unemployed and 1 per cent are

Table 10.9 Women in manual work, by ethnic group

Ethnic group	Skilled	Semi-skilled	Unskilled
All (%)	2.7	9.4	7.2
White (%)	2.7	9.2	7.3
Black (Caribbean) (%)	2.2	12.7	7.8
Black (African) (%)	1.6	9.0	11.9
Black (other) (%)	2.2	9.4	4.2
Indian (%)	3.4	23.7	3.3
Pakistani (%)	3.2	19.8	1.9
Bangladeshi (%)	3.5	17.2	2.5
Chinese (%)	0.5	3.4	4.7
Other Asian (%)	1.6	9.4	6.4
Other (%)	1.6	7.1	3.0

Source: derived from OPCS (1993b) Table 16

Table 10.10 Women in professional and managerial work, by ethnic group

Ethnic group	Employers/ managers in large establishments	Employers/ managers in small establishments	Professional workers	Total
All (%)	3.2	7.5	1.9	12.6
White (%)	3.2	7.6	0.9	12.7
Black (Caribbean) (%)	3.0	3.8	1.0	7.8
Black (African) (%)	3.1	4.5	3.8	11.6
Black (other) (%)	4.3	6.2	1.7	12.2
Indian (%)	1.9	7.1	4.7	13.7
Pakistani (%)	1.6	9.2	3.8	16.6
Bangladeshi (%)	1.3	4.3	5.1	11.7
Chinese (%)	1.9	14.8	10.0	26.7
Other Asian (%)	2.6	5.1	5.1	12.8
Other (%)	4.4	7.8	4.4	16.6

Source: derived from OPCS (1993b) Table 16

on government training schemes. Black Caribbean women are more likely to be in the labour force (83 per cent), they are underrepresented as part-time workers (21 per cent) and more likely to be unemployed (14 per cent) or on a government training scheme. African and other Black women follow the same pattern, though they are slightly less likely to be in the labour force and more likely to be unemployed or on a training scheme than Caribbean women.

Indian women are also more likely to be employed (82 per cent) and less likely to work part-time (24 per cent) than White women, but less so than Black women. They are also more likely than White women to be recorded as unemployed or to be on a government training scheme. Other Asian women follow a similar pattern, including Chinese women – though the Chinese women are more likely than any other ethnic group except White women to work part-time (34 per cent) and also the least likely apart from White women to be recorded as unemployed (8 per cent) or to be on a government training scheme (2 per cent).

Pakistani and Bangladeshi women are less likely than any other ethnic group to be economically active (32 and 24 per cent respectively). However, of those in employment a relatively high proportion work full-time (73 per cent for both groups). These two groups are also the most likely to be recorded as unemployed (35 and 30 per cent respectively) or to be on government schemes (8 and 5 per cent respectively).

The pattern of labour market participation for all women shows a concentration of them in routine non-manual work and semi- and unskilled manual work. However, there are some interesting variations between women from different ethnic groups. Given that a high percentage of economically active women are White it is not surprising that the pattern of their participation dominates the statistics and resembles the overall pattern. Caribbean women are underrepresented as employers and managers, professional workers and 'own account' manual workers and overrepresented as intermediate non-manual workers and semi-skilled manual workers, compared to the overall norm. Black African women are also underrepresented in professional and managerial work and in intermediate and junior non-manual work, and overrepresented in employed professional positions, personal services and unskilled manual work. Other Black women more nearly follow the overall pattern but are slightly overrepresented as employers and managers in large establishments and underrepresented in unskilled manual work.

Indian women, on the other hand, are overrepresented in professional work and skilled, semi-skilled and own account manual work. They are underrepresented as managers and employers in large establishments, routine non-manual work and unskilled manual work. Pakistani women's distribution across the labour market is very similar to that of Indian women, as is that of Bangladeshi women, except that they are overrepresented in personal service work. Other Asian women (except those of Chinese origin) are also overrepresented in professional work and in intermediate non-manual and personal service work; they are underrepresented in skilled and unskilled manual work. Chinese women are overrepresented in all categories of non-manual work and in 'own account' manual work, but underrepresented in all other categories of manual work. (See Table 10.11.)

In terms of the Registrar General's Classification of Social Class, a majority of employed women are classified as 'non-manual' – 68 per cent – and this is true of all ethnic groups, but with some variation. Women are significantly underrepresented compared with men in Social Classes I and II, but, with the exception of Black Caribbean and Black 'other' women, women from non-White ethnic groups are more likely than White women to fall into Social Class I. Black women and 'other' Asian women are more likely than White women to be in Social Class II, while Indian,

Table 10.11 Women's labour market distribution, by ethnic group

Socioeconomic group	White (%)	Caribbean (%)	Black African (%)	Black other (%)	Indian (%)	Pakistani (%)	Bangladeshi (%)	Chinese (%)	Other Asian (%)
Employers/ managers:									
1 Large establishments	3	3	3	4	2	2	1	2	2
2 Small establishments	8	4	4	6	7	9	4	15	5
Professional:									
3 Self-employed	*	*	*	*	1	1	1	1	1
4 Employed	2	1	3	2	4	3	4	7	4
Other non-manual:									
5 Intermediate	18	28	24	20	12	13	16	19	24
6 Junior	37	32	27	38	33	32	31	22	31
7 Personal services	8	8	11	9	3	5	14	16	11
Manual:									
8 Forewomen/ supervisors	1	1	*	1	1	1	*	*	*
9 Skilled	3	2	2	2	3	3	4	1	2
10 Semi-skilled	9	13	9	9	24	20	17	3	9
11 Unskilled	3	8	12	4	3	2	2	5	6
12 Own account	3	1	2	2	7	9	4	9	3

Source: derived from OPCS (1993b) Table 16

Bangladeshi and Pakistani women are notably less likely. If we combine these two classes, Bangladeshi women are significantly less likely than White women to fall in them (25 per cent), while Chinese (38 per cent), 'other' Asian (36 per cent), Black African (34 per cent) and Black Caribbean (34 per cent) are overrepresented here. Well over a third (39 per cent) of employed women are in Social Class IIINM, and this is the modal class for all ethnic groups. However, all ethnic groups except White (39 per cent) and Black 'other' (40 per cent) are underrepresented in this class, with Black Africans being the most underrepresented (28 per cent) (see Table 10.12)

Just over 30 per cent of employed women are in the manual classes. A majority of these are in the 'semi-skilled' class (Class IV), with Black African (34 per cent), Black 'other' (36 per cent), Indian (35 per cent) and Bangladeshi (38 per cent) women being overrepresented in the manual classes as a whole. Women are underrepresented in 'skilled' manual work, compared with men, but Chinese women are notably overrepresented and Bangladeshi women slightly overrepresented in the skilled manual class – Class IIIM – in both cases mainly because of their overrepresentation in 'own account' manual work. Bangladeshi (27 per cent), Indian (27 per

Table 10.12 Women's ethnic group by social class, percentaged by ethnic group (females aged 16+, employed and self-employed)

Social class:	I	II	IIINM	IIIM	IV	V	Armed forces	Not stated
All women (%)	2	28	39	7	16	7	*	1
White (%)	2	28	39	7	16	7	*	1
Black (Caribbean) (%)	1	33	32	6	18	8	*	2
Black (African) (%)	4	30	28	7	16	12	*	3
Black (other) (%)	*	29	40	7	14	4	2	2
Indian (%)	5	24	34	6	27	3	*	7
Pakistani (%)	4	26	33	6	25	3	–	4
Bangladeshi (%)	5	20	30	8	27	2	–	8
Chinese (%)	8	30	31	12	13	5	–	2
Other Asian (%)	5	31	33	7	16	6	–	2
Other (%)	4	34	36	5	13	5	*	2

Key to classes:

I	Professional etc.	IIIM	Skilled, manual
II	Managerial and technical	IV	Partly skilled
IIINM	Skilled, non-manual	V	Unskilled

Not stated: not stated or inadequately described
Source: derived from OPCS (1993b) Table 16

cent) and Pakistani (20 per cent) women are overrepresented in Class IV – semi-skilled manual work. Black African women are overrepresented in Class V – unskilled manual – and Asians and Chinese are underrepresented.

This analysis of labour market positions of economically active women substantiates the view that women are disadvantaged in the labour market and concentrated in a narrow range of occupational groups. While the pattern of distribution across groups varies for women from different ethnic backgrounds, there is no evidence from this statistical analysis that employed non-White women are systematically more disadvantaged than White women. However, non-White women, especially those from Asian ethnic groups, are significantly more likely to be recorded as unemployed in the Census than White women, suggesting discrimination in labour market recruitment, with women from Black and Asian ethnic groups experiencing considerably more difficulty in obtaining employment than White women. Furthermore, it should be noted that this type of analysis does not permit control for factors such as the relationship between educational qualifications and occupational category, or indeed the 'unpicking' of precise occupational position within the broad occupational categories of the Census, so that significant forms of discrimination must necessarily be invisible to it.

References

Abbott, P. A. and Sapsford, R. J. (1987) *Women and Social Class*. London: Tavistock.
Brown, C. (1984) *Black and White Britain: The Third PSI Survey*. Aldershot: Gower.

DOE (Department of Employment) (1991) Ethnic origins and the labour market. *Employment Gazette*, February: 59–72.

DOE (Department of Employment) (1993) Ethnic origins and the labour market. *Employment Gazette*, February: 25–43.

Hakim, C. (1979) *Occupational Segregation*, DOE Research Paper No. 9. London: Department of Employment.

OPCS (Office of Population Censuses and Surveys) (1984) *Census 1981: Economic Activity – Great Britain*. London: HMSO.

OPCS (Office of Population Censuses and Surveys) (1993a) *Census 1991: Report for Great Britain*. London: HMSO.

OPCS (Office of Population Censuses and Surveys) (1993b) *Census 1991: Ethnic Group and Country of Birth*. London: HMSO.

Sly, F. (1994) Ethnic groups and the labour market. *Employment Gazette*, May: 147–59.

Smith, D. J. (1976) *The Facts of Racial Disadvantage: A National Survey*. London: Political and Economic Planning.

Smith, D. J. (1977) *Racial Disadvantage in Britain*. Harmondsworth: Penguin.

Smith, D. J. and McIntosh, N. (1974) *Racial Disadvantage in Employment*. London: Political and Economic Planning.

Appendix A: Women's ethnic and occupational groups in the 1991 Census

Table A1 Women's ethnic group by occupational group, percentaged by ethnic group (females aged 16+, employed and self-employed)

Occupational group:	1.1 (%)	1.2 (%)	2.1 (%)	2.2 (%)	3.0 (%)	4.0 (%)	5.1 (%)	5.2 (%)	6.0 (%)	7.0 (%)	8.0 (%)	9.0 (%)	10.0 (%)	11.0 (%)	12.0 (%)	13.0 (%)	14.0 (%)	15.0 (%)	16.0 (%)
All women	<0.1	3.2	1.8	5.7	0.3	1.6	17.0	1.3	36.7	8.5	0.7	2.7	9.4	7.2	2.9	0.1	0.1	0.5	0.1
White	<0.1	3.2	1.8	5.8	0.3	1.6	16.9	1.4	36.8	8.5	0.8	2.7	9.2	7.3	2.8	0.1	0.1	0.5	0.1
Black (Caribbean)	<0.1	3.0	0.3	3.5	0.1	0.9	26.0	1.0	32.3	8.1	0.7	2.2	12.7	7.8	0.9	<0.1	<0.1	<0.1	0.1
Black (African)	<0.1	3.1	0.6	3.9	0.4	3.4	23.7	0.6	27.4	11.4	0.4	1.6	9.0	11.9	2.2	<0.1	<0.1	0.1	0.4
Black (other)	<0.1	4.3	0.8	5.4	<0.1	1.7	18.8	0.9	38.3	8.9	0.6	2.2	9.4	4.2	2.2	<0.1	<0.1	0.2	1.2
Indian	0.1	1.8	3.4	3.7	1.0	3.7	11.0	0.9	33.2	3.3	0.6	3.4	23.7	3.3	6.6	<0.1	<0.1	0.1	<0.1
Pakistani	<0.1	1.6	5.5	3.7	1.1	2.7	12.3	0.7	32.4	5.1	0.6	3.2	19.8	1.9	9.0	<0.1	<0.1	<0.1	<0.1
Bangladeshi	<0.1	1.3	1.8	2.5	1.0	4.1	15.9	<0.1	31.1	14.2	0.3	3.5	17.2	2.5	3.8	<0.1	<0.1	0.3	<0.1
Chinese	<0.1	1.9	9.3	5.5	0.7	7.3	18.9	0.3	22.0	16.0	0.3	0.5	3.4	4.7	9.2	<0.1	<0.1	0.1	<0.1
Other Asian	0.1	2.6	1.5	3.6	1.0	4.1	22.8	0.9	30.8	11.1	0.3	1.6	9.4	6.4	3.0	<0.1	<0.1	0.1	<0.1
Other	<0.1	4.4	1.2	6.6	0.5	3.9	22.2	1.2	35.0	8.2	0.6	1.6	7.1	4.1	3.0	<0.1	0.1	0.2	0.4

Key to column headings:

Employers and managers in central and local government, industry, commerce etc. – large establishments
  1.1 Employers
  1.2 Managers

Employers and managers in central and local government, industry, commerce etc. – small establishments
  2.1 Employers
  2.2 Managers

  3.0 Professional workers – self-employed
  4.0 Professional workers – employees

Intermediate non-manual workers
  5.1 Ancillary workers
  5.2 Forewomen and supervisors – non-manual

  6.0 Junior non-manual workers
  7.0 Personal service workers
  8.0 Forewomen and supervisors – manual
  9.0 Skilled manual workers
  10.0 Semi-skilled manual workers
  11.0 Unskilled manual workers
  12.0 Own account workers, other than professional
  13.0 Farmers – employers and manager
  14.0 Farmers – own account
  15.0 Agricultural workers
  16.0 Armed forces

Source: derived from OPCS (1993b) Table 16

Table A2 Women's ethnic group by occupational group, percentaged by occupational group (females aged 16+, employed and self-employed)

Occupational group:	All women (%)	1.1 (%)	1.2 (%)	2.1 (%)	2.2 (%)	3.0 (%)	4.0 (%)	5.1 (%)	5.2 (%)	6.0 (%)	7.0 (%)	8.0 (%)	9.0 (%)	10.0 (%)	11.0 (%)	12.0 (%)	13.0 (%)	14.0 (%)	15.0 (%)	16.0 (%)
White	96.0	90.2	96.7	94.6	97.2	91.7	92.5	96.7	97.4	96.5	96.5	96.8	96.4	93.7	97.0	94.1	99.9	99.9	99.0	95.1
Black (Caribbean)	1.1	–	1.1	0.2	0.6	0.4	0.6	1.6	0.7	1.0	1.0	1.0	0.9	1.4	1.1	0.3	–	–	0.2	0.3
Black (African)	0.3	–	0.3	0.1	0.2	0.3	0.6	0.4	0.1	0.2	0.4	0.2	0.2	0.3	0.4	0.2	–	–	0.1	0.6
Black (Other)	0.2	0.7	0.3	0.1	0.2	0.1	0.2	0.2	0.1	0.2	0.2	0.2	0.2	0.2	0.1	0.2	–	–	0.1	2.9
Indian	1.3	6.2	0.7	2.4	0.8	4.2	2.9	0.8	0.9	1.2	0.5	1.0	1.7	3.7	0.6	2.9	–	–	0.4	–
Pakistani	0.2	–	0.1	0.6	0.1	0.8	0.3	0.1	0.1	0.2	0.1	0.2	0.2	0.4	0.1	0.6	–	–	0.2	–
Bangladeshi	<0.1	<0.1	–	<0.1	<0.1	<0.1	<0.1	<0.1	<0.1	<0.1	0.1	<0.1	0.1	0.1	<0.1	<0.1	–	–	<0.1	–
Chinese	0.2	–	0.2	1.4	0.2	0.6	1.2	0.3	<0.1	0.2	0.5	0.1	0.1	0.1	0.2	0.9	0.1	0.1	<0.1	–
Other Asian	0.3	2.9	0.3	0.3	0.2	1.2	0.9	0.5	0.2	0.3	0.4	0.2	0.2	0.4	0.3	0.4	–	–	0.1	0.2
Other	0.3	–	0.5	0.2	0.4	0.6	0.8	0.4	0.3	0.3	0.3	0.2	0.2	0.3	0.2	0.3	–	–	0.2	0.8

Key to column headings: see end of Table A1

Source: derived from OPCS (1993b) Table 16

POSTSCRIPT

The last chapter illustrates an important point about the nature of research interpretation – that one can understand statistics only within a matrix of other understandings. On the face of it the figures seem to show that there are at least some women who do not experience discrimination in the job market. This conclusion might seem to arise from the simple comparison of women of different ethnic groups who are in employment, looking at the average grade of their employment, if we did not take other factors into account. However, in the first place we need to look also at the pattern of employment and unemployment and the extent to which different groups tend towards full- and part-time working. Taking these into account, in the light of known cultural variation in family ideology, gives us more of a picture of how family controls constrain women's entry into the labour market and the position they are able to take within it. Second, to make fair comparisons we would need to be sure we were comparing like with like, and we cannot tell from these figures the extent to which the groups may have differed in, for example, educational qualifications. It is entirely possible that the most 'advantaged' group in this analysis may have suffered some degree of discrimination in comparison with White women, when the level of their qualifications is taken into account. Finally, the classification of jobs is a crude one, and we cannot be sure that the 'professional and managerial' jobs in which some Asian groups seem to be overrepresented are entirely comparable with the jobs in the same categories which are held by the White women. In other words, the figures do not speak for themselves but have to be interpreted by the 'research imagination' in the light of the totality of our other knowledge; it is this which enables us to know what alternative explanations need to be eliminated from the argument.

Another way in which imagination must be exercised, in the interpretation of all the research studies in this book, is in taking account of the extent of procedural reactivity in the study – the extent to which the way in which it is carried out may determine the results, and the extent to which the results may be specific to that particular structured situation. On the whole we think of experiments as the most reactive, followed by surveys, open interviewing, and then participant observation (particularly covert observation, where the researcher is not known to other participants as a researcher). The laboratory experiment is quite clearly a 'game' with rules, and nothing like ordinary life outside the laboratory. The structured survey is a little more like an ordinary-life event, a conversation, but it is still a very artificial conversation, and 'being interviewed' is again a game whose rules we know quite well. 'Open' interviewing is more naturalistic still, but there is still a degree of structure in the conversation, and the fact that the informants know that they are 'undergoing research' makes the situation to some extent artificial. The most naturalistic form of research is participation, where one becomes or passes as a natural participant, and this is the only style which can make serious claims to observing what goes on in real life, independently of the research context. (Its countervailing drawbacks are that it is very time-consuming, very hard and stressful work for the researcher and very dependent for its interpretation on the researcher's understanding of the situation.) The dimension of artificiality is not quite as clear-cut as we are suggesting here; a field experiment – the introduction of an experimental regime into one hospital but not another, for example – might be more naturalistic than some forms of open interviewing. Nor is it necessarily the case that the artificiality of the research situation makes it impossible to generalize results to 'real life'. The reader needs to consider each study on its merits, however, in the knowledge that the very structures which make the research interpretable may also diminish its generalizability.

In this last section we have looked at experiments and quasi-experimental comparisons whose logic mimics that of the experiment except for lack of control over the 'experimental manipulation' (being a smoker or a non-smoker, in the Doll and Hill chapter, or being of a particular ethnic group in the chapter by Abbott and Tyler). This is the most highly structured kind of research design, and its structure puts it in a position to demonstrate causal connections (in experiments) or at least to suggest their presence very strongly (in quasi-experimental studies). It is important to note what they cannot do, however. A structured study of this kind is very good for testing hypotheses, but not good at all for generating theory. In the true experiment the only factors which can emerge as explanatory variables are the experimental manipulation itself or possibly a measured extraneous factor (an alternative explanation which the experiment fails to eliminate). There is no way of telling that some other kind of factor might have been more productive as an explanation, and no way of testing whether the whole explanatory framework is appropriate. An experiment about the effects of working environment on productivity (the Hawthorne study, mentioned earlier) can demonstrate that the environment does or does not have an effect, or that some personal or historical characteristic of the research subjects is a better explanation, but it cannot reframe the question in terms of gender or class or the prevailing economic conditions. Correlational surveys, with less internal structure, are better for thinking round a problem and exploring it; you can collect data on a wide range of variables and look to see what correlates with what, fishing for significant patterns. The power of the study is still limited by the nature of the data collected, however; you cannot analyse what you did not collect, so the study is limited to what you already knew was important or thought might be. 'Open' techniques – open interviewing, and even more participant observation – give much more scope for the unexpected to arise as important. Even here, however, the data collected will be limited by the preconceptions of the researcher, however much he or she may try to guard against this. We must resign ourselves to the fact that theory is not generated, in the last resort, from the results of research, but from the imagination of the researcher. Empirical research is for testing theory or exploring ideas, but the ideas are not themselves a product of the research.

As we have suggested throughout this book, research is very much an act of mind, the adoption of a certain kind of imagination. A double and contrary kind of imagining is required. On the one hand, it is essential to become immersed in the topic area and the people who encapsulate it. You need to be able, to the small extent that this is possible, to think the thoughts of the participants and understand what they take for granted and why, in order to come to a realistic understanding of 'what is going on'. At the same time you need to remain marginal to the action, to the extent that your research design permits, so that you do not disturb the natural scene more than is necessary, and to the perspectives of the participants, so that you can understand what they themselves perhaps do not understand by coming as a stranger to what they take for granted. This double marginality is a counsel of perfection and not possible of achievement, but trying to achieve it is the essential basis both of good research and of an informed understanding of other people's research.

This double marginality is particularly difficult to achieve when the research is concerned with your own place of work and your own professional practice. We have a 'stake' in the results, and we have to live afterwards in the place which we have analysed, both of which make for difficulties. More important, we are deeply enmeshed in the culture and expectations of the workplace and work practices; that which we are exploring and to which we are trying to remain marginal is our own lives and taken-for-granted ways of proceeding. To the extent that we succeed in marginalizing ourselves with respect to these, there is a terrible risk that we may remain marginalized – that the analysis and rethinking involved in research will unfit us for practice at our previous level. Nonetheless we would assert that all good practice is informed by the same kind of imagination that informs research; unexamined practice loses direction and ceases to be able to accommodate change. We therefore commend this book and the whole research enterprise to you, hoping that it does for you what it does for us – that it opens up possibilities and casts some doubt on previously undoubted certainties. Whatever else it does, we hope this book demonstrates that social research is not something arcane, the private preserve of highly trained technicians, but something we can all do for ourselves.

AUTHOR INDEX

SUBJECT INDEX

PSYCHOLOGY FOR NURSES AND THE CARING PROFESSIONS
Sheila Payne and Jan Walker

- What is psychology and how is it relevant to health care practice?
- What influences do psychological factors have in determining outcomes in health care?
- What are the different approaches within psychology which can be used to understand normal human functioning?

Psychology for Nurses and the Caring Professions is one of a series of texts which provide coherent and multi-disciplinary support for all professional groups involved in the provision of health and social care. It introduces students to a range of psychological theories and research, supported by evidence from health psychology. Applications are offered within a variety of health care settings, with an emphasis on health promotion and preventive care.

The authors draw upon their clinical, teaching and research experience to engage the student's interest through the use of case examples, special research-based topics and exercises for group discussion or individual study. The text has been carefully designed with the student in mind: a comprehensive reference list is provided at the end of the book, together with a glossary of terms. The text is illustrated throughout with diagrams, tables and graphs and suggestions for further reading are given at the end of each chapter.

Psychology for Nurses and the Caring Professions is a key textbook for all students undertaking diploma or degree level courses in nursing, health and social care.

Contents
Introduction to psychology – Understanding health and illness – Self-concept and body image – Theories of learning: developments and applications – Perception, memory and patient information-giving – Stress and coping: theory and applications in health care – Development and loss in social relationships – Pain – Social processes in health care delivery – Epilogue – Glossary – References – Index.

240pp   0 335 19410 9 (Paperback)   0 335 19411 7 (Hardback)